MONTH OF MEALS 4
A MENU PLANNER

Published by the American Diabetes Association

AF530801

Cover photo:
Dinner 11

Copyright © 1993 American Diabetes Association®, Inc.

All rights reserved.

No part of this publication may be reproduced or transmitted in any form or by any means, electronic or mechanical, including duplication, recording, or any information storage and retrieval system, without the written permission of the American Diabetes Association.

ISBN 0-945448-28-7

TABLE OF CONTENTS

ACKNOWLEDGMENTS

This publication was created by a committee of the Council on Nutritional Science and Metabolism of the American Diabetes Association (ADA). The committee members were Robin Ann Williams, MA, RD, CDE (Editor); Marti Chitwood, RD, CDE, CN; Ruth Kangas, RD, CDE; Carolyn Leontos, MS, RD, CDE; and Susan L. Thom, RD, LD, CDE. Staff members of the ADA National Center also contributed to this publication, in particular Christine B. Welch, Sherrye Landrum, Stacey N. Wages, Peter Banks, and Susan H. Lau.

Most of the recipes were developed by the committee members who worked on *Month of Meals 4*. A few recipes first appeared in *Diabetes Forecast*, ADA's monthly magazine on living better with diabetes. The recipe for Cauliflower Cheese Soup was developed by Ruth McGary and appears in *The Healthy HomeStyle Cookbook*, published by the ADA. The recipes for Schinkennudelin and Jagerschnitzel were used with permission from Dominica Uhlig. The recipe for Russian Cabbage Roll-Ups was used with permission from Lydia Gaponiuk.

For information on ordering *Month of Meals*, *Month of Meals 2*, *Month of Meals 3*, or *The Healthy HomeStyle Cookbook* or joining the ADA, call the ADA National Center at 1-800-232-3472 or contact your state ADA affiliate, listed in the white pages of the phone book.

People with diabetes can eat a wide variety of foods—including packaged foods, such as frozen entrees—as long as their overall diet is well balanced. Therefore, as a convenient aid to readers who want fast yet healthy meal choices, *Month of Meals 4* includes many brand names or product names. The use of selected brand names does not imply that they are the only brands in a product category suitable for people with diabetes. In addition, although every attempt was made to ensure that these packaged foods meet calorie restrictions of individual menus, the ADA does not endorse these products or guarantee that they are appropriate for all people with diabetes. Consumers are encouraged to read food labels carefully and to consult with a health-care professional to decide whether a food is appropriate for their meal plans.

Photo at right:
Breakfast 5

INTRODUCTION

Welcome to *Month of Meals 4*. This book is designed to help you choose healthy foods easily and quickly. There are complete menus for breakfast, lunch, dinner, and snacks. *Month of Meals 4* is set up in a way that will allow you to mix and match meals for a month or more.

You will find many menus that can be prepared quickly, menus with favorite family dishes, meatless menus, and menus emphasizing low-fat and high-fiber foods. For those who cook for just one or two, there are tips on coping with recipes that make more food than you need for one meal.

Each day's menu—breakfast, lunch, dinner, and a snack—provides approximately 1500 calories. This figure can be adjusted up or down to meet your specific calorie requirements. A day's menus will provide about 45 to 50 percent of the calories from carbohydrate, 20 percent from protein, and about 30 percent from fat.

Month of Meals 4 allows you to choose tasty menus that meet the 1990 *Dietary Guidelines for Americans* (U.S. Dept. of Agriculture and U.S. Dept. of Health and Human Services, Home and Garden Bulletin 232). These menus will help you:

- **Eat a variety of foods.** Eating a wide variety of different foods helps to ensure that you get all the essential vitamins, minerals, and nutrients your body needs. Variety also helps keep your interest so that your diet doesn't become boring. With *Month of Meals 4*, you don't just have one month of daily menus, you can mix and match over 20,000 combinations of breakfasts, lunches, and dinners.
- **Maintain a healthy weight.** *Month of Meals 4* allows you to add and subtract snacks to get just the right calorie intake for you to achieve and maintain a healthy body weight.
- **Choose a diet low in fat, saturated fat, and cholesterol.** *Month of Meals 4* menus average less than 300 milligrams of cholesterol per day and less than 30 percent total fat. Menus emphasize choosing reduced-fat or low-fat foods.
- **Choose a diet with plenty of vegetables, fruits, and grain products.** These foods not only add variety to your diet, but when unprocessed or unrefined, they are an important source of fiber. Unrefined foods are close in form to what Mother Nature gives us, and the closer, the better. In *Month of Meals 4*, high-fiber meals are indicated by
- **Use sugars only in moderation.** These recipes are low in sugar. No-sugar and low-sugar fruit spreads (jams and jellies) are recommended. Simple desserts containing limited amounts of sugar are included. Instead of sugar, you can also use artificial sweeteners that have essentially no calories, such as aspartame (Equal or NutraSweet), acesulfame-K (Sweet One or Sunette), and saccharin (Sweet 'n Low, Sugar Twin, or Sweet 10). The best artificial sweeteners to use when baking are those made of saccharin or acesulfame-K.
- **Use salt and sodium only in moderation.** Most of the menus use salt very moderately. Those menus containing higher than recommended sodium levels are noted for occasional use. Also remember that about one-third of the sodium in your diet comes from the salt shaker. The National Institutes of Health recommends a daily intake of 1,100 to 3,300 milligrams of sodium—eating three healthy meals a day will easily provide this without using the salt shaker. Gradually cut back on the salt you add at the table and in your cooking so your taste buds have time to adjust to a lower level of sodium. If sodium is reduced gradually, you will hardly notice the change

THE SIX FOOD GROUPS

The menus in *Month of Meals 4* have been developed using a meal-planning system that divides foods into six groups: Starch/Bread, Meat and Meat Substitutes, Vegetables, Fruit, Milk, and Fat. Foods are placed into one group or another based on their nutrient make-up of carbohydrate, protein, fat, and calories.

1

Starch/Bread. This group includes whole grains (brown rice, bulgur wheat, wheat berries, oats, barley), cereal, pasta, rice, breads, starchy vegetables (potatoes, corn, lima beans, and winter squashes such as acorn and spaghetti), crackers, and many snack-type foods.

2

Meat and Meat Substitutes. This group includes beef, pork, lamb, veal, poultry, fish, seafood, eggs, tofu, cheese, cottage cheese, and peanut butter. The list divides these foods into lean, medium-fat, and high-fat choices.

3

Vegetables. The vegetable list is made up of nonstarchy vegetables that are either raw or cooked, such as broccoli, asparagus, green beans, cabbage, carrots, salad greens, onions, tomatoes, and summer squashes like crookneck and zucchini.

4

Fruit. This list includes all varieties of fruit—fresh, frozen, canned, and dried—as well as fruit juices.

5

Milk. Included here are milk plus yogurt and buttermilk.

6

Fat. Here you find obvious fats like margarine, butter, cooking oils, mayonnaise, and salad dressings plus other high-fat foods like avocados, olives, nuts and seeds, bacon, sour cream, and cream cheese.

For a complete listing of foods and portion sizes in the six food groups, see *Exchange Lists for Meal Planning,* available from the American Diabetes Association or The American Dietetic Association, or contact a registered dietitian.

Food Group	**Per Serving**			
	Calories	Carbohydrate (grams)	Protein (grams)	Fat (grams)
Starch/Bread	80	15	3	trace
Meat and Substitutes				
Lean	55		7	3
Medium Fat	75		7	5
High Fat	100		7	8
Vegetables	25	5	2	
Fruit	60	15		
Milk				
Skim	90	12	8	1
Low Fat	120	12	8	5
Whole	150	12	8	8
Fat	45			5

INTRODUCING PLANNED-OVERS

You usually cook for one or two people, but all of your favorite recipes make six or eight servings. What should you do with the rest of the servings? The answer is to make planned-overs. Making planned-overs, or planning ahead with leftovers, is a great way to save steps in preparing meals and will also help you and your family follow a healthy eating plan.

Any of the recipes in *Month of Meals 4* that make more servings than you need can become planned-overs. If you're following the recipe for Old-Fashioned Pot Roast (page 65), which makes eight servings, but only need two servings, portion the remainder of the cooked meat (after you remove the fat) into six servings. Undercook about three-quarters of the vegetables; they will finish cooking as you reheat, and nothing says "leftovers" more than mushy vegetables. Package the meals, adding two ounces of gravy on top of each, for the freezer. A dinner portion consists of about 3 ounces of cooked meat (the size of a deck of cards), 2/3 to 1 cup of starch, 1 cup of vegetables, 1 serving of fruit, and a total of 2 fats. If your planned-over isn't totally complete, plan to add fresh foods when you serve it, such as fresh fruit for dessert and a green salad with 1 tablespoon of dressing.

When deciding how to store the servings, think about how you'll reheat them. The most convenient way is to store planned-overs in the same container you will use to reheat. Aluminum foil is great for a conventional oven but doesn't work in a microwave. If you like to use the microwave, make sure you use a microwavable as well as freezer-safe container. Another method is to store each portion in a freezer storage bag and reheat it in another dish once it's thawed. You can thaw the meals quickly in the microwave (but be sure to use the defrost cycle or you will overcook the outside while the inside of the food remains frozen), or set them in the refrigerator the night before or first thing in the morning to thaw.

It's tempting to let your future planned-overs sit cooling on the stove while you eat. However, bacteria grow quickly at warm and room temperatures. It's best to pack and store your planned-overs before you start to eat your meal. (This also cuts down on the temptation to have a little more after you eat.) Foods cool more quickly when refrigerated in small shallow containers versus large containers, reducing the chance of spoiled food.

Once you've put planned-overs in the freezer or refrigerator, don't forget them! Keeping foods too long in the freezer leads to taste loss; if they sit too long in the refrigerator, you risk food spoilage. The pot roast planned-over above will last about 2 to 3 months in the freezer without taste loss but only about 3 to 4 days in the refrigerator without spoiling. Check the Safe Food Storage chart on page 11 when storing your planned-overs.

Because every microwave is a little bit different, experiment when thawing and reheating. If you're not sure how long it will take to reheat, remember that it is easy to put food back in the microwave for another minute. If you overcook, you can't go back.

Breads and muffins should be loosely wrapped in a napkin or microwave-safe paper towel. Keep the wrapping on the bread for a bit after you've taken it out of the oven—this keeps the steam inside the bread instead of letting it escape. One muffin will heat in about 20 seconds; if you have two, don't double the time—30 seconds will do nicely. Overheating breads in the microwave makes them tough (see chart). You may also want to try heating breads on a low or defrost setting for a longer time to avoid chewiness. When you have several frozen muffins or rolls, arrange them in a circle and rotate or turn them over halfway through the cooking time.

Microwaving Breads in Seconds

	Room temperature (Full power)	Frozen (Power level: defrost 30%)
Bread slices		
2	10 to 20	20 to 30
4	20 to 30	30 to 40
6	30 to 40	60 to 80
Rolls, buns, bagels, biscuits, and muffins		
1	20 to 24	60 to 80
2	24 to 30	90 to 100
3	30 to 40	100 to 110
4	40 to 50	60 to 75
6	60 to 90	90 to 120

Be sure to wrap breads in a napkin or microwave-safe paper towel.

After this small amount of planning ahead, you start to reap the benefits:

- Meals, in a healthy portion size, are ready when you are.
- Your meal can be eaten without the temptation of having seconds.
- Preparing and portioning ahead can help strengthen your resolve to follow your meal plan.
- Some foods, especially soups and those in a sauce or gravy, simply taste better in a day or two, when you've given the seasonings time to blend.
- You can enjoy most recipes even though you only need one or two servings at a time.

Planned-overs work for desserts, lunches, and snacks, too.

- The Veggie Pizza (Lunch 5) serves four, but it also makes a great 170-calorie snack. Freeze it in waxed paper, so it's ready in minutes by microwaving.
- One cup of the Lentil Veggie Soup in Lunch 8 also serves as a 170-calorie snack. Freeze 1-cup portions for snacks or 1 1/2-cup portions for lunches.
- One English Pancake (Breakfast 17) is a 60-calorie snack. Cooked pancakes can be placed in stacks with sheets of waxed paper between each pancake and then stored in an air-tight container or freezer bag. (Make sure you remove as much air as possible before you seal the bag or container to avoid freezer burn.) Pancakes can be refrigerated for about 4 days or frozen for up to 6 months. The microwave is great for defrosting or reheating pancakes; just be sure not to overdo them. Add cream cheese filling when you're ready to eat.
- For a 125-calorie snack, try one slice of Low-Fat Lemon Cheesecake (Lunch 13). Individual slices will keep in the refrigerator 3 days.
- To turn Chicken and Rice Bake (Dinner 26) into a lunch-size portion, use 2/3 cup of the rice mixture and half of a chicken breast half or one thigh or one leg. General guidelines for lunch portions are about 2 ounces of meat or cheese, 2/3 to 1 cup of starch, and 1/2 to 1 cup of nonstarchy vegetables. For combination meals, such as zucchini lasagna or a stir-fry, a lunch portion is about three-fourths of the dinner portion.
- The recipe for Bean Muffins in Breakfast 15

makes 24—store those you don't eat within a couple of days in a large freezer storage bag, then remove and microwave them individually as you want them. Let them warm to room temperature on the kitchen counter or defrost in the microwave, then warm them in a preheated conventional oven for several minutes.

Safe Food Storage

Food	Refrigerator (Days at 40°F)	Freezer (Months at 0°F)
FRESH		
Beef roast	3 to 5	6 to 12
Pork roast	3 to 4	4 to 8
Pork chops	3 to 5	3 to 4
Ground hamburger and stew meats	1 to 2	2 to 3
Pork sausage	1 to 2	1 to 2
Chicken pieces	1 to 2	9
Turkey pieces	1 to 2	6
Fish	1 to 2	6
COOKED		
Meat and meat dishes	3 to 4	2 to 3
Poultry covered with broth or gravy	1 to 2	6
Poultry in pieces	3 to 4	1
Poultry dishes	3 to 4	4 to 6
Turkey sausage	1 to 2	1 to 2
Gravy and meat broth	1 to 2	2 to 3
Luncheon meats	3 to 5 (once opened)	1 to 2
Bacon	7	1

Adapted from *The Safe Food Book*, U.S. Dept. of Agriculture, Washington, DC, U.S. Govt. Printing Office, p. 14 (Home and Garden Bulletin 241). For more information on safe food handling, call the National Center for Nutrition and Dietetics at (800) 366-1655 or the U.S. Department of Agriculture at (800) 535-4555.

HEALTHY MEATLESS MEALS

As you flip through the menus in *Month of Meals 4*, you'll find many lunches and dinners that don't include meat. Most people wonder whether leaving meat out of meals is unhealthy. Because animal products contain the most protein per bite, you may be concerned about getting enough protein without eating meat. But consider these facts:

• American adults generally eat more protein than they need. The average woman requires about 45 to 50 grams of protein each day and the average man about 55 to 60 grams. Compare this to the fact that one 8-ounce boneless chicken breast or steak has almost 60 grams of protein.

• The protein in meat often comes "prepackaged" with a lot of fat.

• You can find high-protein foods other than meat in the Meat group: tofu, peanut butter, eggs, and low-fat cheeses.

• Lentils, peas, and beans contain enough protein to be counted as a Lean Meat.

• Foods in the Vegetable, Starch/Bread, and Milk groups all supply protein. On average, 1 Milk serving contains 8 grams of protein, 1 Starch/Bread serving about 3 grams, and 1 Vegetable serving about 2 grams compared to 7 grams of protein in each Meat serving.

• Unlike foods in the Vegetable, Starch/Bread, and Fruit groups, there is no fiber in foods from animals (see "Fiber," page 13).

• The idea that certain foods need to be eaten together at the same meal to supply adequate protein has gone out of date. Eating a variety of foods each day will ensure that you receive all the amino acids (building blocks of protein) necessary for good health, even without meat.

Many people are eating less meat. About 7 percent of Americans describe themselves as vegetarian or as eating plant-based diets. Some reasons are to cut down on fat and calories, to save money, to avoid chemicals sometimes added by the meat growers (although chemical-free or "natural" meats are available), and to avoid that "heavy" feeling after a meal.

Diets without meat have been linked to a reduced risk of developing obesity, non-insulin-dependent or type II diabetes, hypertension, heart disease, kidney disease, and colon cancer. Many studies have pointed out the potential benefits of eating a diet low in protein. For instance, a diet limiting protein to the recommended 45-55 grams per day may slow damage to the kidneys. Health organizations such as The American Dietetic Association believe that vegetarian diets are healthy when appropriately planned.

In the meatless meals in *Month of Meals 4*, the Meat servings have been used as eggs, cheese, tofu, or peanut butter. Cooked beans, lentils, and peas are used as meat substitutes —in the exchange system, 1 cup of these provides 2 Starch/Bread servings and 1 Lean Meat serving. If you have questions about changing your meal plan to include more meatless meals, consult a registered dietitian.

Month of Meals 4 invites you to try the following meatless meals:
Lunches 1, 5, 6, 8, 9, 11, 12, 14, 15, 16, 17, 19, 24, 25, and 28; and
Dinners 4, 6, 8, 9, 11, 20, and 24. And when you choose meatless main dishes, you'll automatically eat less fat (unless you pile on the cheese or add extra fat) and more fiber.

FIBER

Throughout *Month of Meals 4*, we have indicated high-fiber foods with this symbol:

There are many reasons to eat more fiber. Studies suggest that eating a fiber-rich diet may help protect against heart disease and certain types of cancer. Also, because high-fiber foods are very filling and generally take a long time to eat, they satisfy the appetite and help with weight control. Fiber may also help to lower blood glucose levels in people with diabetes.

Fiber is found only in plant products. It is the part of plant foods that we cannot digest or absorb: the outer layer or skin, seeds, leaves, and structural support such as roots. The fiber in plants is divided into two basic types.

Soluble fiber dissolves in water during digestion and forms a gel in the intestinal tract. This material binds bile acids in its gel structure, which may help lower cholesterol and slows down the absorption of certain nutrients, including glucose. This is why eating soluble fiber may be of special benefit to people with diabetes.

Soluble fiber is found in all fruits, vegetables, and grains, but it is particularly rich in starches such as beans, peas, lentils, oats, barley, corn, and sweet and white potatoes; fruits such as citrus fruits, bananas, plums, peaches, pears, apples, apricots, and strawberries; and vegetables such as broccoli, carrots, beans, and zucchini.

Insoluble fiber is the supporting structure of the plant and outer coating such as wheat bran. It does not dissolve in water in the intestinal tract. Instead, it draws water to its surface and causes food to travel through the intestines quickly. This type of fiber is most helpful in treating constipation and diverticulosis and may reduce risk of colon cancer. Insoluble fiber is found in all fruits, vegetables, and grains but is particularly abundant in starches such as whole-grain breads and cereals, brown rice, bulgur, wheat germ and bran, popcorn, potato skins, corn, and peas; the skin and seeds of fruits; and nuts.

Both types of fiber are important for good nutrition and can be easily incorporated into your meal plan. To increase fiber in your diet, keep in mind these recommendations.

- Get half of your daily calories from high-carbohydrate foods like fruits, grains, pastas, cereals, and vegetables. Meats and dairy products do not contain dietary fiber.

- Eat a variety of fiber-rich foods. Your diet should include both soluble and insoluble fiber.

- Eat foods in their most "natural" state whenever possible: fruits and vegetables with their skins, whole-grain flour instead of white flour, brown rice instead of white rice, and whole fruits instead of fruit juice.

- Use breads, cereals, crackers, and flour made primarily from whole grains such as whole wheat, whole oats, and any other whole grains.

- Eat more raw fruits and vegetables. Eat the skins whenever possible.

- Drink plenty of water and other sugar-free fluids. Because fiber draws water into your intestinal tract, you need to drink a lot of fluids so your body can eliminate properly. (Too much fiber and not enough water can cause constipation.)

- Increase your fiber intake gradually. The sudden addition of a lot of fiber can cause intestinal gas, cramping, and diarrhea.

HOW TO USE THIS BOOK

Month of Meals 4 allows you to choose the calorie level that best meets your needs. First, however, you need to know about how many daily calories you require. The best way to do this is to meet with a registered dietitian or certified diabetes educator who can design a meal plan with the right number of calories for your nutritional needs.

Basic Meal Plan
1500 Calories a Day

Each breakfast, each lunch, and each dinner in *Month of Meals 4* has about the same number of calories, so you can mix and match them to suit your own tastes. One day's breakfast, lunch, and dinner is about 1350 calories. By adding two 60-calorie snacks OR one 125-calorie snack, your daily total will be 1500 calories—the Basic Meal Plan. Choose any menus you like. All the portions on the menus are for one person, so you can have everything listed.

If you need more or fewer calories than the basic 1500-calorie menus provide, no problem. Adjusting meals to meet your requirements is as easy as following the instructions on the next few pages.

Basic Meal Plan Plus

If you are following a meal plan that allows you 1800 calories a day, use the chart below to adjust the Basic Meal Plan.

First, choose any menu in *Month of Meals 4* that you want. Then, move down the 1800-calorie column and follow the directions. Breakfast, lunch, and dinner are the same as in the Basic Meal Plan. The extra calories come from snacks—a 125-calorie morning snack, a 125-calorie afternoon snack, and a 170-calorie evening snack.

The chart also shows you how to reach a 2100-calorie meal plan. You may want to alter this plan to meet your needs if you are pregnant or breastfeeding.

	BASIC MEAL PLAN 1500 CALORIES	1800 CALORIES	2100 CALORIES
Breakfast	Total calories: **350**	Same as Basic Meal Plan Total calories: **425**	Add one Meat OR one Starch/Bread to the Basic Meal Plan
Morning Snack		Add one 125-calorie snack Total calories: **125**	Add one 60-calorie snack Total calories: **60**
Lunch	Total calories: **450**	Same as Basic Meal Plan Total calories: **450**	Add one Starch/Bread AND one Fat to the Basic Meal Plan Total calories: **575**
Afternoon Snack		Add one 125-calorie snack Total calories:**125**	Add one 125-calorie snack Total calories: **125**
Dinner	Total calories: **550**	Same as Basic Meal Plan Total calories: **550**	Add one Starch/Bread AND one Milk to the Basic Meal Plan Total calories: **720**
Evening Snack	Two 60-calorie snacks OR one 125-calorie snack Total calories: **125**	Add one 170-calorie snack Total calories: **170**	Add one 170-calorie snack Total calories: **170**

Basic Meal Plan Minus*

If you are following a meal plan that allows you 1200 calories a day, use the chart below to adjust the Basic Meal Plan.

First, choose any menu in *Month of Meals 4* that you want. Then, move down the 1200-calorie column and follow the directions: Eliminate one starch or one milk for breakfast from the Basic Meal Plan. Eliminate one fruit at lunch from the Basic Meal Plan. Eliminate one fat at dinner from the Basic Meal Plan. There are no snacks in the 1200-calorie meal plan.

This chart shows you how to reach a 1200- and a 1350-calorie meal plan.

*To meet your body's most basic nutrient needs, you need to eat at least 1200 calories a day.

	1200 CALORIES	1350 CALORIES	BASIC MEAL PLAN 1500 CALORIES
Breakfast	Eliminate one Starch/Bread or one Milk from Basic Meal Plan Total calories: 270	Same as Basic Meal Plan Total calories: 350	Total calories: 350
Morning Snack			
Lunch	Eliminate one Fruit from Basic Meal Plan Total calories: 390	Same as Basic Meal Plan Total calories: 450	Total calories: 450
Afternoon Snack			
Dinner	Eliminate one Fat from Basic Meal Plan Total calories: 505	Same as Basic Meal Plan Total calories: 550	Total calories: 550
Evening Snack			Two 60-calorie snacks OR one 125-calorie snack Total calories: 125

Sample Meal Plan #1
Here's how to adjust the Basic Meal Plan (1500 calories) for about a 1200-calorie diet.

Meal		Calories	
Breakfast		350	
Plus or minus	-1 Starch/Bread serving(s) (# / type of serving)	-80	Subtotal 270
Lunch		450	
Plus or minus	-1 Fruit serving(s) (# / type of serving)	-60	Subtotal 390
Dinner		550	
Plus or minus	-1 Fat serving(s) (# / type of serving)	-45	Subtotal 505
		TOTAL DAILY CALORIES	1165

Sample Meal Plan #2
Here's how to adjust the Basic Meal Plan (1500 calories) for about a 2200-calorie diet.

Meal		Calories	
Breakfast		350	
Plus or minus	+1 Starch/Bread serving(s) (# / type of serving)	+80	Subtotal 430
Lunch		450	
Plus or minus	+1 Fat serving(s) (# / type of serving)	+60	
	+1 Fruit serving(s) (# / type of serving)	+45	Subtotal 555
Dinner		550	
Plus or minus	+1 Starch/Bread serving(s) (# / type of serving)	+80	
	+1 Med-Fat Meat serving(s) (# / type of serving)	+75	
	+1 Fat serving(s) (# / type of serving)	+45	Subtotal 750
Snacks *(Morning, Afternoon, and/or Evening)*		125	
	+2 Starch/Bread serving(s) (# / type of serving)		
	+2 Milk or Meat serving(s) (# / type of serving)	340	Subtotal 465
		TOTAL DAILY CALORIES	2200

Your Meal Plan

Meal — **Calories**

Breakfast ________

Plus or minus

____ ________serving(s) ________
\# (type of serving)

Subtotal________

Morning Snack

Plus or minus

____ ________serving(s) ________
\# (type of serving)

Subtotal________

Lunch

Plus or minus

____ ________serving(s) ________
\# (type of serving)

____ ________serving(s) ________
\# (type of serving)

Subtotal________

Afternoon Snack

Plus or minus

____ ________serving(s) ________
\# (type of serving)

Subtotal________

Dinner ________

Plus or minus

____ ________serving(s) ________
\# (type of serving)

____ ________serving(s) ________
\# (type of serving)

____ ________serving(s) ________
\# (type of serving)

Subtotal________

Evening Snack

____ ________serving(s) ________
\# (type of serving)

Subtotal________

TOTAL DAILY CALORIES________

HOW TO USE THIS BOOK

Like the first three books in the Month of Meals series, the pages in this book are divided into thirds so that each menu (breakfast, lunch, or dinner) appears on a separate segment. You can either follow each day's meal plan in sequence or flip back and forth between the various menus for added variety.

For example, on one day you may have Breakfast 25, Lunch 5, Dinner 17, and 125-calorie Snack 12 for a total of 1500 calories.

Note that the menus high in fiber are flagged as to help you make higher fiber choices.

Many recipes in this book yield more than the one serving called for in the menus. The total number of servings (yield) and the single serving size are listed at the top of each recipe. The section titled "Introducing Planned-Overs" (page 9) explains how to use extra portions for future meals. Save time and money by taking advantage of planned-overs.

The recipes in this book use these standard abbreviations:

Tbsp. = tablespoon
tsp. = teaspoon
oz. = ounce
lb. = pound

Tips for Healthy Eating

You may:

- use commercial (canned, dry, or frozen) or homemade soups with these menus, but note that they are usually high in sodium, so choose reduced-fat and reduced-sodium varieties.

- use no-sugar or low-sugar fruit spreads (jams or jellies). Limit yourself to 1 to 2 teaspoons (less than 20 calories) per serving.

- use 1 tablespoon of regular salad dressing or 2 tablespoons of reduced-calorie salad dressing interchangeably. Salad dressings that contain less than 6 calories per tablespoon can be used more liberally.

- have raw vegetables on some menus, which can include salad greens and moderate servings of carrot or celery sticks, tomatoes, cucumbers, green peppers, radishes, and the like.

- use butter-flavored granules, such as Butter Buds or Molly McButter, to season vegetables, potatoes, rice, or noodles.

- add your choice of calorie-free beverages, such as coffee, hot or iced tea, mineral water, diet sodas, and sugar-free flavored seltzers.

- measure meat portions after cooking. Four ounces of uncooked meat shrinks to about 3 ounces (about the size of a deck of cards) after cooking.

- season recipes with your favorite spices. Try basil, dill, lemon pepper, paprika, fresh herbs, and fresh garlic or garlic powder. Be sure to choose low-salt varieties when mixtures are purchased.

Photo at right:
Lunch 21

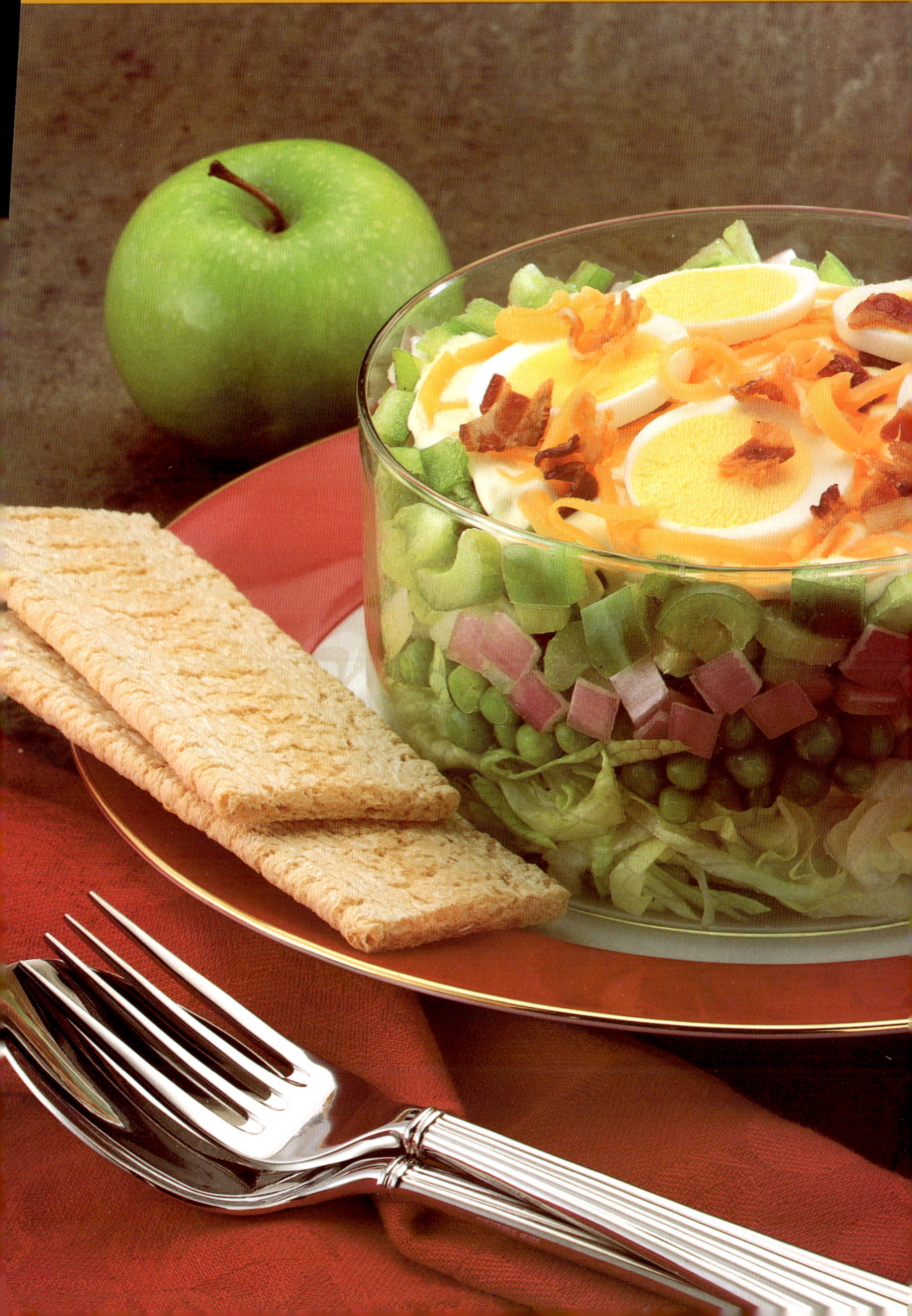

Each **breakfast** in this section has about 350 calories and includes:

2	Starch/Bread	servings
1	Fruit	serving
1	Skim Milk	serving
1	Fat	serving

In some menus, one Meat serving has been used in place of either the Skim Milk serving or one of the Starch/Bread servings.

Each **lunch** in this section has about 450 calories and includes:

2	Starch/Bread	servings
2	Meat	servings
0-1	Vegetable	serving
1	Fruit	serving
1	Fat	serving

In some menus, one Milk serving has been used in place of either one of the Meat or one of the Starch/Bread servings.

Each **dinner** in this section has about 550 calories and includes:

2	Starch/Bread	servings
3	Meat	servings
1-2	Vegetable	servings
1	Fruit	serving
2	Fat	servings

In some menus, one Milk serving has been used in place of either one of the Meat or one of the Starch/Bread servings.

1

Quesadillas:

Nonstick vegetable cooking spray

2 6-inch flour tortillas

2 oz. reduced-fat cheddar cheese, grated

1/4 cup salsa

1 cup carrot sticks

Coat skillet with vegetable spray then heat. Put 1 tortilla in pan and sprinkle with grated cheese. Cover with second tortilla. Brown on both sides.

2

Green salad:

- 1/3 cup kidney beans
- 1 cup other vegetables
- 2 oz. turkey

1 Tbsp. fat-free salad dressing
1 Yogurt Fruit Bar **(see Breakfast 18)**
1 orange

3

1 serving PAN-BROILED SHRIMP
1 medium tomato, sliced
1 cup stone-ground grits
3/4 cup fresh pineapple

PAN-BROILED SHRIMP

Yield: 3 servings/Serving size: 1/3 recipe

Ingredients

1 tsp. margarine
1/3 medium sweet onion, sliced
1/3 lb. shrimp, peeled and deveined
Lemon juice, salt, and pepper to taste

Method

1. Heat margarine in medium saucepan.
2. Saute onion until translucent.
3. Add shrimp. Saute until pink, about 3-5 minutes.
4. Add lemon juice, salt, and pepper to taste.

LUNCH

4

Crabmeat Salad Roll:

1 large hamburger bun

2 oz. imitation crab meat (pollack) chunks mixed with

1 Tbsp. reduced-calorie mayonnaise

1-2 Tbsp. plain nonfat yogurt

Onion and celery, diced, to taste

Lettuce and tomato if desired

1 nectarine

5

1/4 VEGGIE PIZZA
15 grapes

VEGGIE PIZZA

Yield: 4 servings/Serving size: 1/4 pizza

Ingredients

1 8-oz. precooked pizza crust
1/3 cup chunky spaghetti sauce
8 oz. low-fat grated mozzarella cheese
1/2 of a 10-oz. package frozen leaf spinach, thawed, drained well, and chopped
1 clove garlic, crushed
2 Tbsp. olive oil
1 medium tomato, sliced thin

Methods

1. Spread sauce on pizza crust.
2. Spread 2/3 of grated cheese on top.
3. Saute garlic and spinich in oil until limp and just tender. Arrange in ring on pizza crust.
4. Sprinkle with remaining cheese. Top with sliced tomatoes.
5. Bake at 400° for 15 minutes.

6

1 cup SPANISH GARBANZO BEANS
1/2 cup sliced cucumbers in red wine vinegar
1/2 cup grapes

SPANISH GARBANZO BEANS

Yield: 2 servings/Serving size: 1 cup

Ingredients

1/2 cup onions, chopped
1 medium green pepper, chopped
2 Tbsp. olive oil
8 oz. tomato sauce
1 1/4 cup cooked garbanzo beans

Method

1. Saute onions and pepper in olive oil. Add tomato sauce. Cook over medium heat 5 minutes.
2. Add garbanzo beans. Cook over low heat for 15 minutes.

7

1 serving SCHINKENNUDELIN
1 slice bread
1 cup sliced cucumbers with
1 Tbsp. reduced-calorie creamy cucumber dressing
15 grapes

SCHINKEN-NUDELIN *Yield: 1 serving*

Ingredients

1 oz. low-fat ham, cubed
1 Tbsp. reduced-calorie margarine
1/2 cup cooked noodles
1 egg, beaten

Method

1. Brown ham cubes in margarine
2. Add noodles and brown
3. Add beaten egg and continue to brown by turning in sections.

8

1 1/2 cups LENTIL VEGGIE SOUP
Green salad with
2 Tbsp. reduced-calorie dressing
1 fresh orange

LENTIL VEGGIE SOUP

Yield: 4 Servings/Serving size: 1 1/2 cups

Ingredients

2 cups dried lentils
1 Tbsp. salt
1/4 cup vegetable oil
2 large carrots, sliced
1 large onion, diced
1 clove garlic, minced
3/4 cup celery, chopped
1 10-oz. package frozen spinach, thawed
6 oz. turkey ham, cubed

Method

1. Wash lentils. Soak overnight in generous amount of water.
2. Add salt and oil to water before soaking. Do not reduce salt or oil because foaming may result, causing a safety hazard in your pressure cooker. Most of the salt and oil will run off when lentils are drained.
3. Drain lentils.
4. Combine all ingredients in pressure cooker and add water to cover by two inches.

(Continued on page 51)

9

1 serving CAESAR'S SALAD
1 cup frozen melon balls (1/2 cantaloupe, 1/2 honeydew)

CAESAR'S SALAD

Yield: 2 servings/Serving size: 1/2 recipe

Ingredients

1 medium head romaine lettuce
Dressing:
1 clove garlic, crushed
1/2 tsp. black pepper
2 oz. smoked anchovies, drained and patted dry
1 egg yolk, hard boiled
4 Tbsp. lemon juice
2 Tbsp. balsamic vinegar
1 tsp. Dijon mustard, prepared
1 tsp. Worcestershire sauce
2 Tbsp. olive oil
1/3 cup Parmesan cheese
Croutons:
4 1-oz. slices Italian bread, cubed
2 tsp. olive oil
1 clove garlic, halved
1 Tbsp. parsley, chopped

(Continued on page 51)

10

Reuben Sandwich:
- 2 slices toasted rye bread
- 1 oz. cooked corned beef, sliced
- 3/4 oz. mozzarella cheese, sliced
- 1 Tbsp. reduced-calorie Thousand Island salad dressing
- 1/4 cup sauerkraut

1/2 cup pears canned in water

Build sandwich, wrap in microwave-safe paper towel, and microwave 15 seconds or until heated.

11

1 serving PINTOS AND POTATOES
1 cup MASTOKHIAR

PINTOS AND POTATOES

Yield: 6 servings/Serving size: 1/6 recipe

Ingredients

1 1/2 cup dried pinto beans
1/2 tsp. salt (optional)
1 potato, peeled and sliced
2 Tbsp. lemon juice
2 Tbsp. olive oil

Method

1. Wash and rinse beans well. Soak beans overnight in enough water to cover.
2. Drain beans and rinse again. Put beans in slow cooker or saucepan and add water to cover by at least two inches. Add salt.
3. If using a slow cooker, also add the sliced potato and cook on low for about 12 hours.
4. If cooking on stovetop, simmer until beans are almost tender, about 2 hours, then add sliced potato. Simmer another 45 minutes.
5. Add lemon juice and oil when serving.

(Continued on page 51)

12

1 Veggie (Soy) or Harvest Burger
  2 oz. patty (cooked weight) on
  Whole-grain bun with
  Mustard, lettuce, and tomato as desired and
  1 Tbsp. reduced-calorie mayonnaise
3/4 cup CABBAGE-FRUIT SLAW

CABBAGE-FRUIT SLAW

Yield: 4 servings/Serving size: 3/4 cup

Ingredients

- 4 oz. unsweetened pineapple tidbits
- 2 cups cabbage, finely shredded
- 1 medium unpeeled apple, chopped
- 3 Tbsp. raisins
- 1 stalk celery, chopped
- 2 Tbsp. reduced-calorie mayonnaise
- 1 Tbsp. nonfat yogurt
- 2 Tbsp. pecans, chopped

Method

1. Drain pineapple, reserving 2 Tbsp. juice.
2. Combine pineapple, cabbage, apple, raisins, and celery.
3. Combine reserved juice, mayonnaise, and yogurt, and add to cabbage mixture.
4. Chill. Top with pecans to serve.

13

1 serving SHRIMP AND PEA SALAD
2 4-inch bread sticks
1 slice LOW-FAT LEMON CHEESECAKE

SHRIMP AND PEA SALAD

Yield: 4 servings/Serving size: 1/4 recipe

Ingredients

1 16-oz. pkg. frozen peas, thawed
1 tsp. dill weed
1/4 cup red onion, chopped
1 cup cooked shrimp, peeled and deveined
2 Tbsp. nonfat mayonnaise
1/2 cup plain low-fat yogurt

Method

1. Mix all ingedients together.

LOW-FAT LEMON CHEESECAKE

Yield: 16 servings/Serving size: 1 slice

Ingredients

Nonstick vegetable cooking spray
1/4 cup graham cracker crumbs
16 oz. light cream cheese
1 cup sugar
2/3 cup egg substitute
1 3/4-2 cups plain yogurt cheese
2 tsp. vanilla
1 tsp. grated lemon peel
1 Tbsp. lemon juice
Sliced oranges, strawberries, kiwifruit for garnish

(Continued on page 52)

1 Bean Burrito:
- 1 6-inch tortilla (flour or corn)
- 1/4 cup canned pinto beans, mashed
- 2 Tbsp. salsa
- 1 oz. cheddar cheese, shredded
- 1 Tbsp. sour cream

1/2 cup fresh pineapple

Spread beans down the center of tortilla. Top with salsa. Microwave for 45 seconds on high. Top with cheese and microwave for 30-35 seconds, until cheese starts to melt. Fold tortilla over center filling and top with sour cream.

15

1 cup SOUTHWESTERN VEGGIE SOUP
1 Banana Smoothie:
- 1/2 banana
- 1 cup skim or 1% milk

Slice peeled banana and place in blender and add milk, then blend until smooth.

SOUTHWESTERN VEGGIE SOUP

Yield:4 servings/Serving size: 1 cup

Ingredients

2 corn tortillas
Nonstick vegetable cooking spray
1/2 tsp. vegetable oil
1/3 cup onion, chopped
1/3 cup bell pepper, chopped
1 clove garlic, crushed
1 1/2 cup frozen corn
1 medium tomato, chopped
1/3 tsp. beef or vegetable bouillon
1/4 tsp. oregano
1 tsp. cornstarch mixed with 1 Tbsp. water
1 Tbsp. fresh cilantro or parsley leaves, chopped
1/4 cup mild salsa
1 cup canned pinto beans
1 cup mozzarella cheese, shredded
1/8 tsp. thyme

(Continued on page 52)

16

1 EGGPLANT SANDWICH
1 Citrus Fizz

Mix 4 oz. orange or grapefruit juice with 12 oz. sparkling water and artificial sweetener to taste. Serve over ice.

EGGPLANT SANDWICH *Yield: 2 servings*

Ingredients

1 Tbsp. olive oil
1/2 cup onion, chopped
1 clove garlic, crushed
1 1/2 cup eggplant, peeled and chopped
1 medium tomato, chopped
Salt and pepper to taste
2 6-inch pita pockets
3 oz. skim-milk mozzarella cheese

Method

1. Heat oil in medium skillet. Saute onion, garlic, and eggplant for 10-15 minutes. Add tomato and continue cooking until eggplant is tender and tomato liquid reduced.
2. Fill pita pockets (place 1/4 mixture in each half). Sprinkle cheese inside pita.
3. Heat in microwave or oven until cheese melts.

17

1 small baked sweet potato
1/2 cup low-fat cottage cheese topped with
2 Tbsp. currants or raisins and
2 Tbsp. chopped walnuts
1/2 cup steamed spinach

LUNCH

18

Tuna Patty Melt:

2 slices toasted whole-wheat bread topped with
1 oz. water-packed tuna mixed with
1 Tbsp. reduced-calorie mayonnaise and
1 slice (3/4 oz.) mozzarella cheese
1 apple, quartered

Build sandwich, wrap in microwave-safe paper towel, and microwave 15 seconds or until cheese is melted.

19

1/2 can condensed cream of asparagus soup diluted with
1 can skim milk
2 saltine crackers
3/4 cup PEACHY RICE PUDDING

PEACHY RICE PUDDING

Yield: 4 servings/Serving size: 3/4 cup

Ingredients

1 1/2 cups reconstituted dried skim milk
1 cup plus 2 Tbsp. instant rice
1 tsp. vanilla
1/2 tsp. cinnamon
1/4-1/2 tsp. nutmeg
1/4 cup raisins
1 cup no-sugar added canned peaches, diced
Artificial sweetener to taste

Method

1. Put skim milk in saucepan and heat over medium heat until milk scalds, stirring constantly.
2. Add rice, cover, and remove from heat.
3. Wait five minutes, then add vanilla, cinnamon, nutmeg, raisins, and peaches.
4. Mixture will be thin. Cover and let stand for at least 30 minutes or until it thickens.
5. If desired, after mixture cools, add artificial sweetener to taste.

20

Marinated chicken breast sandwich on
1 slice whole-grain bread with
Sliced tomato
Alfalfa sprouts
1/8 medium avocado
1/3 cantaloupe

Marinate chicken breasts in low-calorie Italian salad dressing in refrigerator for 12 hours. Remove from marinade. Broil approximately 3 minutes on each side until done. Slice diagonally. Use 2 oz. chicken for each sandwich.

21

1 serving SEVEN-LAYER SALAD
2 pieces Wasa Crisp Bread
1 medium Granny Smith apple

SEVEN-LAYER SALAD

Yield: 2 servings/Serving size: 1/2 recipe

Ingredients

3 cups iceberg lettuce
1 cup frozen green peas, thawed
1/4 cup onions, chopped
1/2 cup celery, chopped
1/4 cup green pepper, chopped
1/4 cup nonfat yogurt
2 Tbsp. reduced-calorie mayonnaise
2 oz. reduced-fat cheddar cheese
2 slices bacon, cooked crisp and drained well
2 medium hard-boiled eggs, sliced

Method

1. In a medium casserole dish, layer lettuce and other vegetables.
2. Mix together yogurt and mayonnaise and spread on the top layer. Top with cheese, crumbled bacon, and sliced eggs.
3. Cover with plastic wrap and refrigerate 8 hours or more.

22

1 small Egg Drop soup (Chinese take-out)
1 medium eggroll
2 plums

23

3 TUNA PUFFS
1/2 cup chilled Marinated Beets
1 1-oz. hard roll with
1 tsp. butter or margarine
1/2 cup sugar-free gelatin with fruit

Marinate cooked, sliced beets in vinegar and artificial sweetener to taste.

TUNA PUFFS

Yield: 2 servings/Serving size: 3 puffs

Ingredients

6 oz. can water-packed tuna
10 round crackers (such as Ritz), crushed
1 egg, beaten
1/4 cup onions, chopped
2 Tbsp. reduced-calorie mayonnaise
Nonstick vegetable cooking spray

Method

1. Preheat oven to 375°.
2. In a medium bowl, mix all ingredients. Shape into 6 medium balls.
3. Place on a baking sheet that has been coated with nonstick vegetable spray.
4. Bake 25-30 minutes or until golden brown.

24

1 whole-wheat pita pocket filled with
- 2 oz. mozzarella cheese, grated
- 1/4 cup tomato, diced
- 1/4 cup onion, diced
- 1/4 cup green pepper, chopped
- 2 Tbsp. sour cream

1 medium peach

25

1 serving SPICY NOODLE SALAD topped with
1/4 cup oriental noodles
1/2 cup mixed citrus sections

SPICY NOODLE SALAD

Yield: 2 servings/Serving size: 1/2 recipe

Ingredients

1 cup spiral pasta
2 medium carrots, grated
1 medium zucchini, shredded
Salt and pepper to taste
2 oz. reduced-fat cheddar cheese
2 oz. Parmesan cheese
Dressing:
1/4 cup reduced-calorie Italian dressing
1 Tbsp. lemon juice
1 tsp. olive oil
2 tsp. horseradish
1 Tbsp. garlic, minced

Method

1. Cook pasta in boiling water according to package directions. Drain.
2. Mix salad dressing ingredients. Set aside.
3. Combine noodles and vegetables. Pour dressing over salad.
4. Chill. Just before serving, mix in cheeses.

1 1/4 cup PINK SALMON SOUP
3/4 cup fresh blueberries topped with
1/4 cup nonfat, artificially sweetened vanilla yogurt

PINK SALMON SOUP

Yield: 4 servings/Serving size: 1 1/4 cup

Ingredients

4 medium potatoes, diced
2 Tbsp. cornstarch
3 cups skim milk
1/2 of a 14 3/4-oz. can pink salmon
1 small onion, chopped
1 Tbsp. margarine
Salt and pepper to taste

Method

1. Boil potatoes for 10 minutes. Drain water.
2. In small bowl, stir cornstarch with a few drops of water to make a smooth paste.
3. Add cornstarch to milk and whisk to remove lumps. When thickened slightly, add potatoes and remaining ingredients.
4. Simmer for 30 minutes.

27

HAM BBQ SANDWICH:

3 Tbsp. commercial **(or see Dinner 18)** BBQ sauce
2 oz. lean ham, shaved
2 oz. bun

Tossed salad with
2 Tbsp. reduced-calorie dressing
1/3 cup canned pineapple

Heat BBQ sauce in small saucepan. Add ham and heat through. Put ham and sauce on bun.

28

1 CHEESY BREAD STICK
1/2 cup chunky spaghetti sauce
Celery sticks filled with
2 Tbsp. reduced-calorie cream cheese

CHEESY BREAD STICK

Yield: 1 serving

Ingredients

2 oz. soft bread stick
1 oz. mozzarella cheese, grated
2 Tbsp. Parmesan cheese
Garlic powder to taste

Method

1. Split bread stick in half lengthwise. Toast under broiler or in toaster oven until lightly browned.
2. Sprinkle with cheeses and garlic powder if desired. Broil until cheese is melted.
3. Heat spaghetti sauce and dip bread sticks in sauce.

27

3/4 cup BEEF SPIRAL STROGANOFF over
1 cup cooked spiral noodles
4-5 tomato slices topped with
Fresh or dried parsley
1 pear

BEEF SPIRAL STROGANOFF

Yield: 6 servings/Serving size: 3/4 cup

Ingredients

1/2 cup onion, chopped
1 green pepper, chopped
2 Tbsp. margarine
1 1/2 lb. lean ground beef, browned and drained
10 3/4 oz. can tomatoes
10 3/4 oz. can cream of mushroom soup
Pepper to taste
1 Tbsp. catsup

Method

1. Saute onion and green pepper in margarine.
2. Add remaining ingredients and heat until bubbles appear. Serve over noodles.

28

1 SAN FRANCISCO SPECIAL sandwich topped with
1/4 cup MUSHROOM SAUCE
1 apple

SAN FRANCISCO SPECIAL

Yield: 1 serving

Ingredients

2 1-oz. slices sourdough bread
2 oz. lean ham
1 1/2 oz. reduced-calorie Swiss cheese, sliced
4 large spinach leaves
1 hard-cooked egg, sliced
1 Tbsp. Parmesan cheese

Method

1. Top one slice of bread with ham, Swiss cheese, spinach, and egg. Cover with mushroom sauce and sprinkle with Parmesan cheese.
2. Broil until light and bubbly and cheeses start to melt. Top with second slice of bread, toasted.

MUSHROOM SAUCE

Yield: 1 serving/Serving size: 1/4 cup

Ingredients

1 tsp. butter or margarine
1/2 cup mushrooms, sliced
1 Tbsp. flour
1/2 cup skim or 1% milk

(Continued on page 54)

1 1/2 cups BRUNSWICK STEW
1 cup salad greens with
1/2 cup citrus sections and

Dressing:
1 Tbsp. orange juice
1 Tbsp. vinegar
2 tsp. vegetable oil

BRUNSWICK STEW

Yield: 4 servings/Serving size: 1 1/2 cups

Ingredients

4 medium chicken thighs, skin and fat removed
2 celery stalks, chopped
1/2 cup onion, chopped
1 28-oz. can tomatoes and juice
1 Tbsp. sugar
1 cup frozen lima beans
1 cup frozen corn
1 cup potatoes, cubed
Salt and pepper to taste

Method

1. Combine first three ingredients plus 1 cup water in a medium saucepan and bring to a boil. Cover and simmer 1 1/2-2 hours.
2. Save the broth. Remove bones and chop chicken. Put chicken in the broth.
3. Add tomatoes, juice, sugar, lima beans, corn, and potatoes. Bring to a boil.
4. Cover, reduce heat, and simmer 30–40 minutes or until vegetables are tender.

DINNER

1 pouch FISH IN PARCHMENT
2/3 cup wild rice pilaf (cook per package instructions but reduce margarine to 1 Tbsp.)

Tossed salad with
2 Tbsp. reduced-calorie Caesar dressing
1/2 grapefruit

FISH IN PARCHMENT

Yield: 2 servings/Serving size: 1 pouch

Ingredients

Nonstick vegetable cooking spray
2 18-inch squares of cooking parchment
1 small tomato, sliced
2 large mushrooms, sliced
1 small green onion, sliced
1/4 cup each carrot and celery strips, julienned
2 4-oz. fish fillets (salmon, halibut, or sole)
Pinch of thyme and summer savory
Drinking straw

Method

1. Coat both sides of parchment squares with vegetable spray and fold each in half.
2. Arrange a bed of vegetables in the middle of one half of each piece of parchment.
3. Place fish on top of vegetables and sprinkle with herbs.

(Continued on page 49)

3

1 serving PRUNE-STUFFED TENDERLOIN
1/2 baked acorn squash with
1 tsp. margarine
5 spears steamed asparagus
Tossed salad with
2 Tbsp. reduced-calorie dressing

PRUNE-STUFFED TENDERLOIN

Yield: 4 servings/Serving size: 1/4 recipe (2 1/2-inch slice)

Ingredients

15 dried pitted prunes, coarsely chopped
1/3 cup chicken broth
1/4 cup celery, chopped
1/4 cup onion, chopped
1 tsp. vegetable oil
3 slices multigrain bread, cubed
1/8 tsp. poultry seasoning
1 lb. pork tenderloin
1 clove garlic, crushed
1/8 tsp. fennel seeds
1/4 tsp. pepper
1/8 tsp. salt
Nonstick vegetable cooking spray
1 Tbsp. margarine

(Continued on page 49)

DINNER

2 shells TOFU MANICOTTI
1 cup FRESH VEGETABLE SALAD
8 oz. artificially sweetened nonfat yogurt with
2 Tbsp. raspberry sauce

Blend 1 cup fresh or frozen unsweetened raspberries with 1/4 tsp. almond extract, 2 packets artificial sweetener, and 1-2 Tbsp. orange liqueur or orange juice. Strain through sieve or cheesecloth to remove seeds if desired.

TOFU MANICOTTI

Yield: 14 servings/Serving size: 2 shells

Ingredients

1 1/4 lb. low-fat cottage cheese
1 lb. tofu, mashed
1 1/2 cups grated Parmesan cheese, divided
1 medium onion, finely chopped
3 Tbsp. parsley, chopped
1/2 tsp. salt
3 eggs, beaten
28 manicotti chells, uncooked
4 cups spaghetti sauce

(Continued on page 49)

1 serving CHICKEN RATATOUILLE
2/3 cup barley
Tossed salad with
2 Tbsp. reduced-calorie dressing
3/4 cup mixed fresh fruit salad, topped with
2 Tbsp. nonfat fruit-flavored yogurt

CHICKEN RATATOUILLE

Yield: 4 servings/Serving size: 1 breast half and 1 1/2 cups of vegetables

Ingredients

4 chicken breast halves, boned, with skin removed
1 Tbsp. olive oil
1 small eggplant, cubed
2 small zucchini, sliced
1 onion, sliced
1/2 lb. mushrooms, sliced
1 green pepper, sliced
1 large tomato, cubed
1/2 tsp. garlic powder
1 tsp. dried parsley
1 tsp. basil
1 tsp. pepper
1/2 cup part-skim mozzarella cheese, grated

(Continued on page 50)

6

1 piece ZUCCHINI LASAGNA
1 cup steamed broccoli with
2 tsp. margarine
1 cup 1% or skim milk
1/2 poached pear with
2 Tbsp. raspberry sauce

ZUCCHINI LASAGNA

Yield: 9 servings/Serving size: 3 x 3-inch piece

Ingredients

Nonstick vegetable cooking spray
1 16-oz. jar marinara sauce
1 8-oz. can tomatoes
1/2 lb. (9-12) curly lasagna noodles
15 oz. ricotta cheese
2 large eggs, beaten
1/4 tsp. dried basil
1/4 tsp. dried oregano
1/4 cup Parmesan cheese
3 cups zucchini, coarsely grated
1/8 tsp. pepper
2 tsp. flour
8 oz. mozzarella, coarsely grated

Method

1. Preheat oven to 350°. Coat a 9-inch square baking dish with vegetable spray.
2. Combine marinara and tomatoes. Spread 1/2 cup of the mixture over bottom of dish. Arrange uncooked noodles in dish, breaking off ends to make them fit. Place ends in open spaces.

(Continued on page 50)

7

1 cup CAULIFLOWER CHEESE SOUP
1 cup MIXED GREENS WITH ORANGE VINAIGRETTE topped with 2 oz. grilled chicken
1 PUMPKIN-CORNMEAL MUFFIN
1 apple

CAULIFLOWER CHEESE SOUP

Yield: 8 servings/Serving size: 1 cup

Ingredients

2 cups potatoes, cut into chunks
3 1/2 cups cauliflowerettes, divided
1 medium carrot, chopped
3 cloves garlic, chopped
1 large onion, chopped
1/2 tsp. salt (optional)
4 cups water or chicken stock
1 1/2 cups low-fat cheddar cheese, grated
3/4 cup 1% milk
1/4 tsp. dill
1/4 tsp. caraway seed
1/4 tsp. dried mustard
Black pepper to taste
3/4 cup buttermilk
8 tsp. scallion, chopped, for garnish if desired

(Continued on page 50)

8

2 slices medium Thin-n-Crispy Pizza Hut vegetable/cheese pizza
2 cups tossed salad with
2 Tbsp. reduced-calorie dressing

1 1/3 cups BLACK BEAN CHILI
1 serving Mixed Greens With Orange Vinaigrette **(see Dinner 7)**
1/2 cup Peachy Rice Pudding **(see Lunch 19)**

BLACK BEAN CHILI

Yield: 6 servings/Serving size: 1 1/3 cups

Ingredients

1 large onion, chopped
1 Tbsp. vegetable oil
1 cup water
2 Tbsp. chili powder
1 tsp. dried oregano
1 28-oz. can tomatoes, undrained, chopped
1 15-oz. can black beans, drained, rinsed
1 7-oz. can sweet corn, undrained
1 6-oz. can tomato paste
1 green pepper, cubed
1 red pepper, cubed
2 oz. (1/2 cup) Monterey Jack cheese, shredded

Method

1. In large saucepan or Dutch oven, cook onion in oil until tender. Add remaining ingredients except cheese.
2. Bring to a boil. Reduce heat, cover, and simmer 30 minutes or until peppers are tender.
3. Top with cheese when serving.

DINNER

(10)

3 oz. FISH CREOLE
2/3 cup rice
1/2 cup green beans
1 peach

FISH CREOLE

Yield: 4 servings/Serving size: 3-oz. fillet plus sauce

Ingredients

4 3-oz. fish fillets
Nonstick vegetable cooking spray
2 Tbsp. lemon juice
2 Tbsp. onion, finely chopped
4 Tbsp. reduced-calorie margarine
1/2 cup green peppers, chopped
1 cup canned tomatoes, chopped
1/2 cup juice from canned tomatoes
Pepper to taste
2 tsp. flour

Method

1. Place fish fillets in baking pan coated with vegetable spray.
2. Mix together lemon juice, onion, and 2 Tbsp. melted margarine.
3. Pour mixture over fish. Heat oven to 350° and bake uncovered or until fish flakes easily with fork.
4. While fish is baking, prepare creole sauce: Saute green pepper in remaining margarine. Add tomatoes, juice, and pepper. Simmer until mixture is heated.

11

2 STUFFED VEGETARIAN PEPPERS
1 cup skim milk
1/2 cup ITALIAN FRUIT SALAD

STUFFED VEGETARIAN PEPPERS

Yield: 6 servings/Serving size: 2 peppers

Ingredients

2 cups uncooked couscous
4 cups boiling water
6 red peppers
6 yellow peppers
1/4 cup shallots, minced
1/4 cup and 1 Tbsp. olive oil
1 lb. asparagus
3 Tbsp. tarragon
2 cups spring peas
1/2 tsp. pepper
1/2 tsp. paprika

Method

1. Place couscous in a large bowl and cover with boiling water. Cover with plastic wrap and let sit for 20 minutes.
2. Slice tops off peppers and remove the white membranes and seeds. Steam peppers and their tops for 5-7 minutes until tender.
3. Saute the shallots in 1 Tbsp. olive oil until translucent. Chop the tips of the asparagus into 1-inch pieces (save the rest for soup).

(Continued on page 51)

DINNER

12

Jagerschnitzel

3-oz. pork tenderloin, browned on each side with
1 Tbsp. reduced-calorie margarine, over
1 cup cooked noodles and topped with
1/4-1/2 cup mushroom gravy

1/2 cup green beans
1 small Baked Apple **(see Dinner 15)**

Prepare mushroom gravy by boiling 1 cup sliced mushrooms 3-5 minutes in 1 oz. package of au jus gravy mix and 2 cups of water.

13

1 serving ORIENTAL CHICKEN
1/3 cup rice or oriental noodles
Tossed salad with
1 tsp. oil and vinegar
3/4 cup FRUIT CRISP
1 cup skim or 1% milk

ORIENTAL CHICKEN

Yield: 4 servings/Serving size: 1/4 recipe

Ingredients

4 chicken thighs, skin and fat removed
2 Tbsp. "lite" soy sauce
1 tsp. brown sugar
1/2 cup celery, sliced
1/4 cup white, yellow, or green onion, chopped
4 oz. (1/2 8-oz. can) water chestnuts, drained and rinsed
8 oz. fresh mushrooms, washed and sliced
1/4 tsp. garlic powder
1/4 tsp. powdered ginger
1/4 tsp. dried red pepper flakes
8 oz. snow peas, fresh or frozen
1 tsp. cornstarch plus 2 Tbsp. cold water

(Continued on page 52)

DINNER

14

3-oz. (cooked weight) cube steak pan fried with
Nonstick vegetable cooking spray and
Worcestershire sauce to taste
1 small dinner roll
1 6-inch corn on the cob with
1 Tbsp. reduced-calorie margarine
Tossed salad with lettuce, tomato, and carrot with
1 Tbsp. reduced-calorie dressing
1 small wedge of watermelon

15

3 PORCUPINE MEATBALLS
1/2 cup steamed carrots
1 cup celery sticks and radishes
10 small Spanish olives
1 BAKED APPLE

PORCUPINE MEATBALLS

Yield: 2 servings/Serving size: 3 meatballs

Ingredients

8 oz. ground beef
1/3 cup uncooked rice
1 1/2 Tbsp. dried minced onion
1/4 tsp. pepper
1/8 tsp. oregano
1 cup tomato sauce

Method

1. Mix meat, rice, onion, and sea sonings until well blended.
2. Form into six equal-size meatballs.
3. Place rack in pressure cooker. Pour tomato sauce and 1 1/2 cups water into cooker. Add meatballs.
4. Cover pressure cooker and place pressure regulator on vent pipe.
5. Heat until cooker reaches optimum pressure. Cook 12 minutes.
6. Remove from heat and let pressure drop of its own accord.

(Continued on page 52)

16

1 serving OVEN CRISPY CHICKEN
1/2 cup POTATO SALAD
1 cup crudities—cherry tomatoes, cauliflower, and broccoli
1 Tbsp. reduced-calorie Ranch dressing
3/4 cup Fruit Crisp **(see Dinner 13)**

OVEN CRISPY CHICKEN

Yield: 8 servings/Serving size: 1/2 breast or drumstick and thigh

Ingredients

1 3- to 3 1/2- lb. chicken, cut up (or purchased parts)
1 Tbsp. canola oil
1/2 cup plus 2 Tbsp. flour
3/4 tsp. seasoned salt (or salt-free seasoning)
1/2 tsp. pepper

Method

1. Disjoint chicken and remove skin and fat. (This is easier if chicken is partly frozen.)
2. Spread oil over bottom of 13 x 9 x 2-inch baking pan.
3. Combine flour and seasoned salt and pepper. Dredge chicken well in this mixture.
4. Place chicken pieces in pan and bake at 400° for 1 hour, turning once.

(Continued on page 53)

17

1 cup SEAFOOD GUMBO
1/3 cup rice
Tossed salad with
2 Tbsp. reduced-calorie French dressing
1 1-oz. slice French bread
1 tsp. margarine
1/2 cup BREAD PUDDING

SEAFOOD GUMBO

Yield: 8 servings/Serving size: 1 cup

Ingredients

2 tsp. olive oil
2 medium onions, chopped
1 cup canned tomatoes
1 clove garlic
1 Tbsp. chopped parsley
1 tsp. ground thyme
2 cups chicken broth
1 lb. orange roughy or other firm, boneless fish
1 cup chopped celery
2 cups frozen okra
1/2 large bell pepper, chopped
12 oz. frozen precooked shrimp
1/4 cup tomato paste

Method

1. Heat pressure cooker.
2. Add oil and saute onions until translucent. Stir in all ingredients except shrimp and tomato paste.
3. Close cover securely, place pressure regulator on vent pipe and bring to pressure on medium-high heat.

(Continued on page 53)

18

1 serving BARBECUED CHICKEN
1 6-inch corn-on-the-cob
1/2 cup broccoli, steamed
1/2 cup carrot sticks
1 slice SALLY LUNN PEACH CAKE

BARBECUED CHICKEN

Yield: 2 servings/Serving size: 1/2 of recipe

Ingredients

2 thighs and 2 legs
1/2 cup BARBECUE SAUCE

Method

1. Marinate raw chicken pieces in barbecue sauce at least 2 hours in the refrigerator, turning occasionally.
2. Cook over outdoor grill until chicken is no longer pink inside. Time will depend on the distance the chicken is from the flame. (Boneless pieces cook more quickly.)

BARBECUE SAUCE

Yield: 4 1/2 cups/Serving size: 1/4 cup

Ingredients

1 small onion, minced
2 8-oz. cans tomato sauce
2 cups water
1/4 cup wine vinegar

(Continued on page 53)

19

1 serving BOK CHOY SAUTE
2/3 cup steamed brown rice
1/3 cup fresh pineapple chunks mixed with
1/2 cup fresh strawberries

BOK CHOY SAUTE

Yield: 2 servings/Serving size: 1/2 recipe

Ingredients

1 Tbsp. sesame or vegetable oil
1 clove garlic, crushed
1 cup shiitake or other mushrooms, sliced
1 1/2 cups bok choy, sliced, with leaves
4 oz. (1/2 8-oz. can) water chestnuts, drained
1 Tbsp. "lite" soy sauce
8 oz. pork tenderloin, thinly sliced

Method

1. Add oil to a large skillet or wok over medium-high heat and cook garlic 1 minute.
2. Add pork, stirring constantly, and cook 3-5 minutes. Add mushrooms and cook, stirring constantly, 1 minute. Add bok choy and water chestnuts and cook, stirring constantly, 2-3 minutes.
3. Add soy sauce; toss to coat.

20

1 serving LENTIL LOAF
1/2 cup Marinated Beets **(see Lunch 23)**
Tossed salad with
2 Tbsp. reduced-calorie dressing
1/2 cup sliced peaches

LENTIL LOAF

Yield: 4 servings/Serving size: 1/4 loaf

Ingredients

1 cup dry lentils
1/2 cup onion, chopped
1/2 cup oatmeal, uncooked
2 eggs, beaten
2 oz. reduced-fat cheddar cheese
2 oz. skim or low-fat mozzarella cheese
1/2 cup tomato sauce
1/2 tsp. oregano
1/4 tsp. basil
1/4 tsp. thyme
Salt and pepper to taste
Nonstick vegetable cooking spray

Method

1. Cook lentils until tender, about 40 minutes.
2. Preheat oven to 350°.
3. Place lentils in a large bowl and mash using a fork or potato masher. Add remaining ingredients and mix well.
4. Place mixture in a loaf pan that has been coated with vegetable spray.
5. Bake 30 minutes until firm.

21

1 serving SAUSAGE AND CORNBREAD PIE
1/2 cup steamed green beans
Tossed salad with
2 Tbsp. reduced-calorie dressing
1 medium pear

SAUSAGE AND CORNBREAD PIE

Yield: 4 servings/Serving size: 1/4 recipe

Ingredients

14 oz. turkey sausage
1 cup onion, chopped
1 clove garlic, crushed
1 28-oz. can tomatoes and juice
1/4 cup green chilies, chopped and undrained
3/4 cup frozen corn
1 tsp. chili powder
Nonstick vegetable cooking spray
2/3 cup cornmeal
1/4 cup whole-wheat or white flour
1 1/2 tsp. baking powder
1/4 tsp. salt
1 egg, beaten
1/3 cup skim or 1% milk
1 Tbsp. corn oil

(Continued on page 54)

22

1 1/2 cups JAMBALAYA
Tossed salad with
2 Tbsp. reduced-calorie dressing
1/4 cup melon cubes

JAMBALAYA

Yield: 4 servings/Serving size: 1 1/2 cups

Ingredients

4 oz. lean ham, chopped
1 cup onion, chopped
2 celery stalks, chopped
1 medium green pepper, chopped
1 28-oz. can tomatoes and juice
1/4 cup tomato paste
1 clove garlic, minced
1 Tbsp. minced parsley
1/2 tsp. minced thyme
2 whole cloves
1 Tbsp. vegetable oil
2/3 cup uncooked white or brown rice
16 medium-large shrimp, peeled and cleaned

Method

1. Thoroughly mix all ingredients except shrimp in a slow cooker. Cover and cook on low setting for 7-10 hours.
2. One hour before serving, turn slow cooker to high setting. Stir in uncooked shrimp. Cover and cook until shrimp are pink and tender.

23

2 skewers of HAWAIIAN KEBABS
2/3 cup steamed rice
Tossed salad with
2 Tbsp. reduced-calorie dressing

HAWAIIAN KEBABS

Yield: 4 servings/Serving size: 2 skewers

Ingredients

1 Tbsp. soy sauce
1/4 cup pineapple juice
1/2 tsp. garlic powder
1 tsp. ground ginger
1/2 tsp. dry mustard
1/4 tsp. pepper
2 Tbsp. corn oil
14 oz. chicken breast, cut into 1-inch cubes
2 cups fresh or juice-packed pineapple chunks
2 medium green peppers, cut in chunks
16 medium mushrooms
8 cherry tomatoes

Method

1. Combine first seven ingredients in a small saucepan and bring to a boil. Reduce heat and simmer 5 minutes. Let cool.
2. Pour mixture into a shallow dish and add chicken, tossing gently to coat. Cover and marinate at least 1 hour in the refrigerator, stirring mix ture occasionally.

(Continued on page 54)

DINNER

24

2 BLACK BEAN CAKES with
1/2 cup CILANTRO SALSA
2 Tbsp. reduced-fat sour cream
1/2 cup frozen yogurt

BLACK BEAN CAKES

Yield: 2 servings/Serving size: 2 cakes

Ingredients

1 1/4 cups black beans, cooked
1/2 cup onion, chopped
1/2 cup cilantro or fresh parsley, chopped
2 Tbsp. Korean chili-garlic paste or plain tomato paste
1 egg
2 Tbsp. skim or 1% milk
Salt and pepper to taste
1/4 cup dry bread crumbs
2 Tbsp. olive oil

Method

1. Thoroughly mix all ingredients except bread crumbs and olive oil. Add bread crumbs to mixture and form into 4 patties.
2. Gently slide patties into an oiled, hot saute pan. Saute until brown and crisp on both sides.

(Continued on page 54)

25

3-oz. turkey cutlet browned with
3 Tbsp. white wine or white grape juice
1 medium baked sweet potato
1/2 cup green beans
2 tsp. margarine
15 grapes

DINNER

26

1 serving CHICKEN AND RICE BAKE
1/2 cup steamed zucchini
1/2 cup pears canned in water

CHICKEN AND RICE BAKE

Yield: 6 servings/Serving size: 1 chicken breast half and 3/4 cup rice mixture

Ingredients

1 cup celery, sliced
3/4 cup onion, chopped
2 Tbsp. margarine
2 Tbsp. parsley, dried
3 cups cooked rice
1 cup cooked sliced carrots
1/4 tsp. salt
1/8 tsp. pepper
Nonstick vegetable cooking spray
3 chicken breasts, split into halves
1 10 3/4-oz. can cream of mushroom soup
1/4 cup milk

(Continued on page 54)

1

3 APPLE FLAPJACKS with
1 1/2 tsp. diet margarine
1 oz. turkey sausage
8 oz. low-calorie cranberry juice cocktail

APPLE FLAPJACKS

Yield: 3 servings/Serving size: 3 4-inch pancakes

Ingredients

3/4 cup sifted flour
1/2 tsp. baking powder
1/4 tsp. cinnamon
1 1/2 tsp. vegetable oil
1 1/2 tsp. sugar
1/4 cup egg substitute
1 cup apple, finely chopped
1/2 cup skim or 1% milk
Nonstick vegetable cooking spray

Method

1. Sift flour with baking powder and cinnamon.
2. Mix oil, sugar, egg substitute, and apple.
3. Combine wet and dry ingredients, gradually adding in milk.
4. Spray a nonstick griddle with vegetable spray.
5. Bake flapjacks on griddle as for pancakes. Sprinkle with brown sugar substitute if desired.

2

1 serving MANGO YOGURT
1 OATMEAL-RAISIN SCONE

MANGO YOGURT

Yield: 6 servings/Serving size: 1 cup

Ingredients

1 large mango, peeled and pitted
1 tsp. vanilla extract
1 cup plain nonfat yogurt
1 pint blueberries
3 bananas, sliced
1/2 pint strawberries, sliced

Method

1. Peel and puree mango and stir in vanilla and yogurt.
2. Arrange mixed fruit decoratively in serving bowls on top of yogurt.

(Continued on page 49)

3

1 Peanut Butter Chocolate Shake
1 slice whole-wheat toast
1 tsp. margarine

Blend 1 cup skim milk, 1/2 frozen banana, 1 Tbsp. peanut butter, and 2 Tbsp. sugar-free powdered chocolate mix.

4

Old-Fashioned Strawberry Shortcakes:

1 3-inch biscuit
1 1/4 cup sliced strawberries
1 cup skim milk
Artificial sweetener as desired

Split biscuit and place half in a bowl. Cover with 1/2 of strawberries, then top with other half of biscuit. Cover with remaining strawberries and pour milk over biscuit and strawberries.

1 serving EASY SPUD BREAKFAST
1 slice whole-grain toast
1 tsp. calorie-reduced margarine
3/4 cup mixed berries

EASY SPUD BREAKFAST *Yield: 2 servings/Serving size: 1/2 recipe*

Ingredients

1 large baked potato with skin
Nonstick vegetable cooking spray
1/4 cup onions, chopped
1/4 cup green or red peppers, chopped
1 oz. lean ham, chopped
1 large egg
2 Tbsp. reduced-calorie cheddar cheese, grated
Fresh or dried parsley

(Continued on page 50)

6

1 PEACHY OAT MUFFIN
1/2 banana
8 oz. fruit-flavored artificially sweetened yogurt

PEACHY OAT MUFFINS

Yield: 18 muffins/Serving size: 1 muffin

Ingredients

2 cups rolled oats (regular or quick cooking)
1 cup whole-wheat flour
2 Tbsp. sugar
3/4 tsp. baking soda
1 1/4 tsp. baking powder
1 egg or 1/4 cup egg substitute
1 1/2 cup plain nonfat yogurt
2 Tbsp. vegetable oil
3/4 cup peaches, sliced, peel on or off
Nonstick vegetable cooking spray

(Continued on page 50)

7

1 cup Wheat Hearts cereal
1 cup 2% milk
2 Tbsp. raisins

8

1 6-inch pita
1/4 cup low-fat cottage cheese
1/2 banana, sliced
1 Tbsp. chopped walnuts

Cut pita in half. Divide cottage cheese and banana between halves and stuff in pockets. Sprinkle with walnuts.

1 slice POPPY SEED COFFEE CAKE
1 fresh peach, sliced, or 1/2 cup juiced-packed peaches
1/4 cup low-fat cottage cheese

POPPY SEED COFFEE CAKE

Yield: 10 slices/Serving size: 1 slice

Ingredients

1 cup buttermilk
1 2-oz. jar poppy seeds
1/2 tsp. almond extract
3 eggs or 3/4 cup egg substitute
1 cup unsweetened applesauce
3 Tbsp. margarine, melted
1 tsp. ground cinnamon
2 1/2 cups whole-wheat flour
1 tsp. baking powder
1 tsp. baking soda
1/2 tsp. salt
1/4 cup white sugar
10 packets Sweet One
Nonstick vegetable cooking spray

(Continued on page 51)

10

Cinnamon Tortilla Pocket:
- 1 6-inch tortilla filled with
- 1/4 cup ricotta cheese blended with
- 1/2 packet artificial sweetener and
- 1/4 tsp. cinnamon

Tropical Fruit Cup:
- 3/4 cup fresh pineapple, mango, kiwi, banana, and/or papaya

Spread mixture down middle of tortilla; fold four corners over into a square and microwave on low for 30 seconds until warm.

11

1 serving LOWCOUNTRY GRITS AND SAUSAGE
1/2 cup fresh citrus sections

LOW-COUNTRY GRITS AND SAUSAGE

Yield: 2 servings/Serving size: 1/2 recipe

Ingredients

2 oz. turkey sausage
1/2 cup uncooked yellow or white grits (stone-ground are best)
2 large eggs, beaten
1/2 cup skim milk
1/2 tsp. thyme, if desired
1/8 tsp. garlic salt, if desired
Nonstick vegetable cooking spray

Method

1. The night before, cook turkey sausage and crumble into small pieces.
2. Cook grits according to package directions.
3. Combine eggs, milk, thyme, and garlic salt in medium bowl. Add a small amount of hot grits and mix well. Add to rest of grits.
4. Mix well and pour into a loaf pan that has been coated with vegetable spray. Cover and refrigerate overnight.
5. Next morning, remove from refrigerator and let stand 15 minutes before baking. Bake at 350° for 45 minutes or until done.

BREAKFAST

12

Breakfast pita:

- 1 6-inch whole-wheat pita pocket, toasted, filled with
- 1/4 cup egg substitute scrambled with
- 1 tsp. margarine
- Chopped onion and green pepper if desired
- 3/4 oz. mozzarella cheese

1/2 cup orange juice

13

2 3-inch biscuits with
2 tsp. no-sugar-added fruit spread
1 medium peach
1 cup skim milk

14

2 slices whole-wheat toast topped with
1 tsp. reduced-calorie margarine and half of a mixture of
1/4 cup low-fat cottage cheese and
1/2 cup sliced fresh strawberries sprinkled with
Artificial sweetener

15

1 BEAN MUFFIN
1 tsp. peanut butter
1 peach

BEAN MUFFIN

Yield: 24 muffins/Serving size: 1 muffin

Ingredients

1 cup pinto beans, canned or precooked
2 cups whole-wheat flour
3/4 cup granulated sugar
2 1/2 tsp. baking powder
1 tsp. each salt and cinnamon
1/2 tsp. each ground cloves and nutmeg
1/2 cup butter or margarine
1 cup skim milk
1 tsp. molasses
1 tsp. grated orange rind
2 eggs, unbeaten
1 tsp. vanilla

(Continued on page 52)

2 Cheese Cornucopias:
- 2 slices bread
- 1 oz. low-fat cheese, grated
- 2 toothpicks
- 1 tsp. soft margarine

1/2 cup orange juice

Trim crusts from bread and sprinkle with cheese. Fold bread to opposite corners and secure with a toothpick. Spread top with margarine. Place on tray in toaster oven at 350° until brown, about 10 minutes. Remove toothpicks to serve.

17

2 ENGLISH PANCAKES
1/2 cup applesauce
1 cup skim or 1% milk

ENGLISH PANCAKES

Yield: 8 pancakes/Serving size: 2 pancakes

Ingredients

1/2 cup flour
1/2 cup whole-wheat flour
1 1/4 cup skim or 1% milk
2 egg whites
Nonstick vegetable cooking spray
1/2 cup fat-free cream cheese
8 tsp. low-sugar jam or jelly

Method

1. Combine flours, milk, and egg whites and beat until smooth.
2. Heat an 8- to 10-inch nonstick skillet that has been coated with nonstick vegetable spray to medium-high.
3. Put 1/4 cup batter into skillet and rotate skillet to spread batter evenly over bottom of pan.
4. Cook for 20 seconds on each side.

(Continued on page 53)

BREAKFAST

18

1 YOGURT FRUIT BAR
1 cup nonfat yogurt or skim or 1% milk

YOGURT FRUIT BARS

Yield: 8 bars/Serving size: 1 bar

Ingredients
1 1/2 cup whole-wheat flour
1 tsp. baking soda
1/2 tsp. baking powder
1 tsp. cinnamon
1/2 tsp. ground ginger
1 6-oz. package mixed dried fruits
1/3 cup chopped walnuts
1 cup nonfat or low-fat plain yogurt
1 large egg
1/4 cup apple juice concentrate
2 Tbsp. vegetable oil
Nonstick vegetable cooking spray

(Continued on page 53)

19

Bacon and Egg Sandwich:
- 2 slices high-fiber bread, toasted
- 1 egg, cooked in nonstick pan
- 1 strip of bacon, cooked crisp

1 medium tangelo

20

Breakfast Parfait:
- 8 oz. nonfat artificially sweetened vanilla yogurt
- 4 chopped pecan halves
- 1/2 banana
- 3 Tbsp. wheat germ

3 graham crackers (2 1/2-inch squares)

Layer parfait ingredients in a parfait glass.

21

1 slice JOHNNYCAKE
1 1/2 tsp. reduced-calorie margarine
2/3 cup raspberries with
Artificial sweetener if desired
1 1/2 oz. turkey ham
4 oz. orange juice

JOHNNY-CAKE

Yield: 1 loaf of 12 slices/Serving size: 1 slice

Ingredients

2 cups corn meal
1 1/2 tsp. salt
1 tsp. baking soda
2 Tbsp. sugar
2 cups buttermilk
1/2 cup egg substitute
2 Tbsp. vegetable oil
Nonstick vegetable cooking spray

Method

1. Mix dry ingredients together.
2. Add buttermilk, egg substitute, and oil.
3. Mix well. Pour into 8 x 10-inch loaf pan coated with vegetable spray.
4. Bake in 400° oven for 30 minutes.

22

1 wedge cantaloupe (1/3 5-inch melon) filled with mixture of
1/4 cup cottage cheese and
2 Tbsp. raisins
6 Wasa Extra Crisp or Light Rye Crisp crackers

23

1 serving BREAKFAST BAKE
Fruit compote:
1/2 cup melon cubes
1/4 cup strawberries

BREAKFAST BAKE

Yield: 2 servings/Serving size: 1/2 recipe

Ingredients

Nonstick vegetable cooking spray
4 pieces whole-grain bread, cut into 1/2-inch cubes
1 oz. extralean ham
1/4 cup green or red pepper, chopped
1/4 cup onion if desired, chopped
1 oz. reduced-calorie cheddar cheese
1 large egg or 1/4 cup egg substitute
1/2 cup skim or 1% milk
1/2 tsp. dry mustard

(Continued on page 54)

24

Hot Granola:

- 1 cup oatmeal mixed with
- 2 Tbsp. raisins
- 2 chopped walnuts
- Artificial sweetener to taste

1 cup skim or 1% milk

1 CARROT-RAISIN MUFFIN
1 cup sweet milk for "dunking":
  1 cup warm skim or 1% milk with
  1/2 tsp. vanilla

CARROT-RAISIN MUFFINS

Yield: 12 muffins/Serving size: 1 muffin

Ingredients

1 cup flour
1/2 cup whole-wheat flour
1 Tbsp. baking powder
1/2 tsp. ground cinnamon
1/4 tsp. salt
2 large eggs
1/2 cup packed light brown sugar
3/4 cup buttermilk
1/4 cup vegetable oil
1 cup carrots, coarsely grated
1/2 cup raisins

(Continued on page 54)

26

1 Healthy Choice Egg Muffin
1/2 cup unsweetened applesauce, mixed with
2 Tbsp. chopped pecans

27

Commuter Breakfast:

- 1 Tbsp. peanut butter
- 1 cup nonfat plain yogurt
- 1/2 banana (or 1/2 cup other fruit)
- 3-4 ice cubes, if desired
- Artificial sweetener, if desired
- 1/3 cup All-Bran cereal

Blend all ingredients in a blender except cereal. Pour in mug, then top with cereal.

BREAKFAST

28

1 serving CREAMED CHIPPED BEEF OVER TOAST
3/4 cup equal parts of berries and melon, cubed

CREAMED CHIPPED BEEF OVER TOAST

Yield: 2 servings/Serving size: 1/2 recipe

Ingredients

2 oz. dried beef
1 Tbsp. flour
1 cup skim or 1% milk
2 tsp. butter or margarine
2 slices whole-wheat bread

Method

1. Pour enough hot water over beef to cover. Soak for 20-30 minutes. Pour off water and slice into strips.
2. Melt butter in a small saucepan. Stir in flour with a wooden spoon until well mixed.
3. Add milk, a little at a time, until all milk is added.
4. Add beef and heat until bubbly.
5. Cut toast in half and pour beef over toast.

Breakfast #2 (Continued)
OATMEAL-RAISIN SCONES
Yield: 12 scones/Serving size: 1 scone
Ingredients
2 cups rolled oats
2 cups flour
1/4 cup sugar
1 tsp. baking powder
1/2 tsp. baking soda
6 Tbsp. chilled margarine
2/3 cup raisins
1 1/4 cup buttermilk
1 Tbsp. skim milk

Method
1. Grind 1 cup oats in food processor. Blend in flour, sugar, baking powder, and baking soda.
2. Add margarine. Blend until mixture resembles coarse meal.
3. Transfer to a large bowl. Add raisins and remaining oats.
4. Make a well in center of mixture and gradually add buttermilk. Knead dough on lightly floured surface, about 10 turns.
5. Divide into 3 pieces. Pat to 3/4-inch thick. Divide each into quarters.
6. Brush with skim milk and bake in preheated oven at 375° for 28 minutes. (After getting scones ready to bake, you can wait up to 4 hours to put them in the oven.)

Dinner #2 (Continued)
FISH IN PARCHMENT
Method
4. Fold the other half of parchment over the top and double fold edges to make an air-tight seal to encase the fish and vegetables.
5. When ready to cook, open the last fold of parchment, insert the end of a drinking straw, and inflate the pouch. Remove straw and quickly reseal the pouch to trap the air.
6. Bake on a baking sheet at 400° for 10-15 minutes.
7. To serve, place pouch on plate and cut an "X" in the top. Peel back four corners.

Dinner #3 (Continued)
PRUNE-STUFFED TENDERLOIN
Method
1. Bring prunes and broth to a boil in a saucepan. Remove from heat and let stand for 10 minutes.
2. Saute celery and onion in oil until tender.
3. Place bread cubes and poultry seasoning in a large bowl. Toss to mix. Add celery, onions, prunes, and broth. Toss lightly to blend. Add more broth if dressing is too dry.
4. Trim excess fat from tenderloin. Cut lengthwise to within 1/2 inch of each end and almost to the bottom, leaving bottom connected. Open out the meat and pound sides of pocket to about 1/4 inch thickness.
5. Combine garlic, fennel seeds, pepper, and salt and rub on the inside of pocket.
6. Spoon stuffing into opening of tenderloin. Press gently to close.
7. Tie tenderloin securely with heavy string at 1-inch intervals.
8. Place tenderloin on roasting rack coated with vegetable spray.
9. Place rack in roasting pan. Insert meat thermometer into thickest part of tenderloin.
10. Place tenderloin in oven preheated to 500°. Immediately reduce temperature to 350°.
11. Cook 20 minutes, then brush on melted margarine and cook an additional 10-15 minutes.
12. Remove from oven, cover with aluminum foil, and let stand 10 minutes before slicing.
13. Slice into 4 equal servings.

Dinner #4 (Continued)
TOFU MANICOTTI
Method
1. Mix together first seven ingredients, except for 1/2 cup Parmesan. Stuff shells with mixture.
2. Pour 1 cup sauce into each of two 7 x 11-inch pans. Place stuffed manicotti on top of sauce and cover with remaining sauce. Cover pans with foil and bake 25 minutes at 350°.
3. Uncover, sprinkle with remaining Parmesan, and bake 5 minutes or until shells are tender.

FRESH VEGETABLE SALAD
Yield: 5 servings/Serving size: 1 cup
Ingredients
4 cups spinach leaves, torn
1 cup cauliflower, chopped
1 cup red cabbage, shredded
1/2 cup mushrooms, sliced
1/2 cup radishes, sliced
Dressing:
2 Tbsp. nonfat dressing
1-2 tsp. Dijon mustard
2 Tbsp. honey
1 Tbsp. tarragon vinegar

Method
1. In large bowl, combine all salad ingredients and toss gently. In small bowl, combine all dressing ingredients using a wire whisk.
2. Pour dressing over salad and toss gently. Serve immediately with coarsely ground pepper.

Breakfast #5 (Continued)
EASY SPUD BREAKFAST
Method
1. Slice baked potato in half the long way. Scoop out 1/3 of the potato pulp (save for another meal). Set shells on a microwave-safe dish.
2. Spray a nonstick skillet with vegetable spray and saute onions and peppers for about 5 minutes or until soft.
3. Add ham and saute another 1-2 minutes. Add the beaten egg and cook until egg is done. Add salt and pepper to taste.
4. Fill each potato half with egg mixture. Top with grated cheese. Heat at 400° in a conventional oven or microwave until hot. Garnish with parsley.

Dinner #5 (Continued)
CHICKEN RATATOUILLE
Method
1. Saute chicken in olive oil about 2 minutes per side.
2. Add eggplant, zucchini, onion, mushrooms, and green pepper. Cook 10 minutes.
3. Add tomato and remaining ingredients, except cheese.
4. Simmer 3-5 minutes more.
5. Arrange chicken breasts on top of vegetables and sprinkle cheese over the breasts. Cook 1 more minute until cheese melts.
6. Serve over barley or rice.

Breakfast #6 (Continued)
PEACHY OAT MUFFIN
Method
1. Mix dry ingredients together.
2. Beat egg; add yogurt, oil, and dry ingredients.
3. Mix enough to dampen flour. Fold in peaches.
4. Coat muffin pan with vegetable spray; fill with batter and bake at 400° for 25 minutes or until done.

Dinner #6 (Continued)
ZUCCHINI LASAGNA
Method
3. Combine ricotta, eggs, basil, oregano, and Parmesan. Spread over lasagna noodles. Top with more noodles and 1/2 cup more sauce.
4. In the same bowl, combine zucchini, pepper, and flour. Spoon into baking dish and spread to make a level layer. Top with more lasagna noodles and remaining sauce.
5. Cover dish with foil and place on a rimmed baking sheet. Bake 55-60 minutes or until noodles are tender. Remove foil and sprinkle with mozzarella. Bake 15-20 minutes more or until cheese is golden brown (or place under broiler). After removing from oven, let stand 15 minutes before cutting.

Dinner #7 (Continued)
CAULIFLOWER CHEESE SOUP, ETC.
Method
1. Cook potatoes, 2 cups cauliflower, carrots, garlic, onion, salt, and liquid for 10 minutes. Turn burner off and let stand for 15 minutes. Puree in blender until smooth and creamy.
2. Heat gently and whisk in cheese, milk, and seasonings.
3. Steam or saute remaining cauliflower and add to soup.
4. Just before serving, whisk in buttermilk. Garnish with scallions.

MIXED GREENS WITH ORANGE VINAIGRETTE
Yield: 8 servings/Serving size: 1 cup with 1 1/2 Tbsp. dressing
Ingredients
1/4 cup white wine vinegar
1/4 cup orange juice
2 packets artificial sweetener
2 Tbsp. onion, finely chopped
1/4 tsp. salt
1/8 tsp. pepper
2 tsp. olive oil
2 tsp. Dijon mustard
3 cups iceberg lettuce, torn
3 cups spinach leaves, torn
2 cups lean cooked ham, cubed
1 cup seedless red grapes, halved
1/4 cup green onions, sliced
1 11-oz. can mandarin orange segments, chilled and drained

Method
1. In jar or blender with a tight-fitting lid, combine first eight ingredients and shake well. Refrigerate one hour.
2. In large bowl, combine remaining ingredients with dressing and toss gently.

PUMPKIN-CORNMEAL MUFFINS
Yield: 12 muffins/Serving size: 1 muffin
Ingredients
1 1/2 cups flour
1/2 cup yellow cornmeal
1 Tbsp. baking powder
1 tsp. salt (optional)
1/2 tsp. ground cinnamon
1/2 tsp. ground nutmeg
1 egg, beaten
1/2 cup canned pumpkin

1/2 cup 1% milk
1/4 cup honey
1/4 cup vegetable oil
Nonstick vegetable cooking spray

Method

1. Stir together first six ingredients.
2. Combine egg, pumpkin, milk, honey, and oil. Add all at once to dry ingredients, stirring just until dry ingredients are moistened.
3. Coat muffin pans with vegetable spray and fill 2/3 full. Bake at 400° for 20-25 minutes.

Lunch #8 (Continued)
LENTIL VEGGIE SOUP
Method

5. Close cover securely. Place pressure regulator on vent pipe and cook for 18 minutes after pressure is achieved.
6. Allow pressure to drop of its own accord.
7. In no case should the contents of the pressure cooker pass the maximum capacity line. Refer to your owner's manual for explanation. Recipe may be halved.

Breakfast #9 (Continued)
POPPY SEED COFFEE CAKE
Method

1. Combine buttermilk, poppy seeds, almond extract, eggs, applesauce, and melted butter.
2. Combine all dry ingredients in a large bowl.
3. Make a well in the center of the dry ingredients. Slowly add mixed liquid ingredients until blended.
4. Pour batter into a 10-inch tube pan that has been coated with vegetable spray.
5. Bake at 350° for about 45 minutes or until done. Cool 10 minutes before removing from pan.

Lunch #9 (Continued)
CAESAR'S SALAD
Method

1. Crisp lettuce by separating leaves and rinsing well under cold water. Pat dry with paper towels and break into 2-inch pieces. Roll in clean paper towels and place in plastic bag and seal. Refrigerate until cold and well crisped, about 1 hour.
2. For dressing, combine garlic, pepper, and anchovies in a blender. At high speed, blend until garlic and anchovies are finely chopped. Add egg yolk, lemon juice, vinegar, mustard, and Worcestershire sauce. Blend until mixture is smooth.
3. Turn blender on high and, with machine running, remove center of lid or lid itself. Slowly pour olive oil in a thin, steady stream. Blend until all oil is added and dressing is smooth and creamy. Set aside or refrigerate until ready to add to salad. Do not leave out of refrigeration for more than 1 hour.
4. For croutons, heat olive oil and garlic in medium skillet until oil is hot and garlic is fragrant. Remove pan from heat and cool to room temperature. Discard garlic.
5. Add the bread cubes and toss to coat. Saute over medium-high heat until golden brown. Cool.
6. To build salad, place crisp lettuce pieces in a medium bowl. Pour dressing over salad and sprinkle with grated Parmesan cheese and croutons.
5. Add flour and simmer until sauce thickens. Pour over fish.

Lunch #11 (Continued)
MASTOKHIAR
Yield: 2 servings/Serving size: 1 cup
Ingredients

1 1/2 cups plain low-fat yogurt
1 cucumber, peeled and finely chopped
1/4 cup raisins
1/8 tsp. salt
1/2 tsp. dried or 1/2 Tbsp. fresh mint leaves, chopped

Method

1. Mix all ingredients.
2. Chill 1 or 2 hours before serving.

Dinner #11 (Continued)
STUFFED VEGETARIAN PEPPERS
Method

4. With a wooden spoon, fluff the couscous and add the shallots, aspargus tips, tarragon,peas, pepper, and 1/4 cup olive oil. Mix thoroughly.
5. Stuff the mixture into the peppers using about 2/3 cup per pepper. Cover with the tops of the peppers. Put the peppers into a large casserole dish with 1/4 inch of water at the bottom. Cover and bake in a preheated oven at 350° for 45 minutes.
6. To serve, discard each pepper top and sprinkle with paprika.

ITALIAN FRUIT SALAD
Yield: 6 servings/Serving size: 1/2 cup
Ingredients

1/4 cup freshly squeezed orange juice
Juice and rind of 1/4 lemon
1 apple, unpeeled, cubed
1 pear, unpeeled, cubed
1/4 lb. seedless grapes
1 peach (if in season), peeled, sliced
1 banana, sliced
2 packets artificial sweetener
1 Tbsp. orange liqueur (optional)

Method

1. Combine orange, grated lemon rind, and lemon juice in a large bowl. As you cut fruit, mix it with juice to keep it from discoloring.
2. Add sweetener and orange liqueur to taste. Toss lightly.
3. Cover bowl with plastic wrap and chill at least 2 hours before serving.

Lunch #13 (Continued)
LOW-FAT LEMON CHEESECAKE
Method

1. Heat oven to 350°. Coat 9-inch springform pan with vegetable spray and sprinkle bottom with graham cracker crumbs. Refrigerate.
2. In a large bowl, beat cream cheese until smooth. Grandually add sugar, beating until smooth. Add remaining ingredients except fruit and beat until smooth. Pour into pan.
3. Bake 50-60 minutes or until edges are set. (To minimize cracking, place shallow pan half full of hot water on lower oven rack while baking.)
4. Remove from oven and cool on wire rack. Remove sides of pan and refrigerate 6 hours or overnight. Top with fruit just before serving.

Dinner #13 (Continued)
ORIENTAL CHICKEN
Method

1. Place 3/4 cup water and all ingredients except snow peas and cornstarch in pressure cooker. Close cover securely. Place pressure regulator on vent pipe and bring to pressure on medium-high heat.
2. Cook 6 minutes with pressure regulator rocking gently.
3. Let pressure drop of its own accord (takes about 10 minutes).
4. Remove cooker lid and add snow peas, return to a boil. Do not cover.
5. Stir in cornstarch mixed with water and simmer until thickened.
6. Serve over rice or oriental noodles.

FRUIT CRISP
Yield: 6 servings/Serving size: 3/4 cup
Ingredients
Nonstick vegetable cooking spray
3 cups sliced apples
1 16-oz. can juice-packed peaches
1/2 cup oatmeal
1/2 cup whole-wheat flour
3/4 tsp. cinnamon
3/4 tsp. nutmeg
3/4 tsp. cornstarch
2 Tbsp. reduced-calorie margarine

Method

1. Lightly coat a 9 x 9-inch baking pan with vegetable spray.
2. Put apples and peaches in pan along with the peach juice.
3. In a separate bowl, combine oats, flour, cinnamon, nutmeg, cornstarch, and margarine. Stir half of mixture into fruit.
4. Sprinkle remainder of the dry mixture over top of the fruit and bake at 375° for 30 minutes.

Breakfast #15 (Continued)
BEAN MUFFIN
Method

1. Preheat oven to 400°. Line muffin tins with baking cups.
2. Mash beans with an electric mixer or potato masher.
3. Sift dry ingredients into a large bowl.
4. Add shortening, 3/4 cup milk, molasses, and orange rind; beat 2 minutes.
5. Add eggs, 1/4 cup milk, vanilla, and mashed beans; beat 2 minutes more.
6. Fill muffin tins two-thirds full. Bake 20 minutes. Cool on wire rack.

Lunch #15 (Continued)
SOUTHWESTERN VEGGIE SOUP
Method

1. Cut tortillas into eighths.
2. Coat nonstick cookie sheet with vegetable spray.
3. Toast tortillas on cookie sheet at 400° for 10 minutes or until crisp.
4. Saute vegetables in vegetable oil for 2 or 3 minutes.
5. Add 2 cups water, bouillon, oregano, cornstarch paste, cilantro, salsa, and beans and let simmer for 5 minutes.
6. Ladle soup into 4 shallow oven-proof bowls.
7. Distribute toasted tortilla pieces equally between the bowls.
8. Top each bowl with 1/4 cup shredded cheese and a pinch of thyme.

Dinner #15 (Continued)
BAKED APPLE
Yield: 2 servings/Serving size: 1 apple
Ingredients
2 small cooking apples
2 tsp. margarine
2 tsp. reduced-calorie currant or grape jelly

Method

1. Core apples, leaving bottom intact.
2. Place in oven-proof baking dish with 1/2 inch water.
3. Put 1 tsp. margarine and 1 tsp. jelly in each apple.

4. Bake at 350° for 30 minutes or until tender.
5. Baste with jelly/margarine mixture before serving.

Dinner #16 (Continued)
POTATO SALAD
Yield: 8 servings/Serving size: 1/2 cup
Ingredients
4 eggs, hard boiled and peeled
1/4 cup reduced-calorie or fat-free mayonnaise
2 Tbsp. skim or 1% milk
1/4 tsp. salt if desired
1 tsp. prepared mustard if desired
2 Tbsp. onion, finely chopped
1 1/2 lbs. white or red new potatoes, boiled in skins

Method
1. Cut one egg in half; remove yolk and place it in a large mixing bowl. Mash egg yolk with a fork.
2. Add mayonnaise, milk, and, if desired, salt and mustard. Mix well.
3. Peel potatoes while they are still warm, and cut into small pieces.
4. Chop remaining egg white and remaining eggs. Add chopped onion.
5. Mix all ingredients well. Chill thoroughly.

Breakfast #17 (Continued)
ENGLISH PANCAKES
Method
5. Treat pan with vegetable spray between each pancake.
6. Place cooked pancakes on warm plate with waxed paper between them.
7. Microwave cream cheese until soft and spreadable (use low or defrost setting).
8. Spread 1 Tbsp. cream cheese and 1 tsp. jam on each pancake and roll up.

Dinner #17 (Continued)
SEAFOOD GUMBO
Method
4. When pressure regulator begins to rock gently, time cooker for 1 minute.
5. Cool cooker at once under running water. Gently stir in tomato paste, then add shrimp (may still be frozen). Bring to a boil.
6. Serve when heated through.

BREAD PUDDING
Yield: 6 servings/Serving size: 1/2 cup
Ingredients
2 1/2 cups bread, cubed
2 cups warm skim or 1% milk
1 cup egg substitute
6 packets artificial sweetener (not aspartame)
1 tsp. vanilla
1/4 tsp. cinnamon
1/4 tsp. nutmeg
3/4 cup raisins
Nonstick vegetable cooking spray

Method
1. Soak bread in warm milk for 15 minutes in large bowl.
2. Combine remaining ingredients except raisins and pour over soaked bread.
3. Add raisins. Stir gently until blended.
4. Coat 6 custard cups with vegetable spray. Pour mixture equally into cups.
5. Place cups in a pan filled with enough water to surround but not spill into cups. Bake in water bath about 45 minutes at 350°.
6. When done, custard should shimmy when pressed gently.

Breakfast #18 (Continued)
YOGURT FRUIT BARS
Method
1. Preheat oven to 350°.
2. In a large bowl, mix all dry ingredients. Add dried fruit and walnuts.
3. Combine yogurt, egg, apple juice concentrate, and oil.
4. Make a well in the center of the dry ingredients and gently mix in the wet ingredients until blended.
5. Coat a 9 x 9 x 13-inch pan with vegetable spray. Spread batter in pan.
6. Bake 45-50 minutes or until done. Cool 10 minutes before slicing.
7. Slice into 8 equal servings. Individual portions freeze well.

Dinner #18 (Continued)
BARBECUE SAUCE
Ingredients
1/4 cup Worcestershire sauce
1 tsp. salt if desired
2 tsp. paprika
2 tsp. chili powder
1 tsp. pepper
1/2 tsp. cinnamon
1/8 tsp. ground cloves

Method
1. Combine all ingredients in saucepan. Bring to a full boil.
2. Reduce heat and simmer for 20 minutes.

SALLY LUNN PEACH CAKE

Yield: 1 loaf of 12 slices/Serving size: 1 slice

Ingredients

2 cups sifted flour
3 tsp. baking powder
1/2 tsp. salt
1 egg, beaten
3/4 cup skim or 1% milk
1/2 cup vegetable oil
1/4 cup sugar
Nonstick vegetable cooking spray
Fresh or juice packed peaches

Method

1. Sift flour with baking powder and salt.
2. Combine egg, milk, and oil in a large bowl. Add sugar. Stir in dry ingredients. Do not overmix.
3. Place in loaf pan that has been coated with vegetable spray.
4. Bake at 375° for 30 minutes.
5. Top each slice with 1/3 cup peaches.

Dinner #21 (Continued)

SAUSAGE AND CORNBREAD PIE

Method

1. Cook sausage, onion, and garlic in a large skillet over medium heat until meat is browned and crumbled.
2. Add tomatoes, chilies, corn, and chili powder, and simmer 20 minutes. Spoon mixture into an 8-inch baking dish that has been coated with vegetable spray. Set aside.
3. Combine cornmeal, flour, baking powder, and salt in a medium bowl, mixing well.
4. Combine egg, milk, and oil in a small bowl. Add to dry ingredients, stirring just until moistened.
5. Spread cornbread mixture over sausage mixture. Bake at 375° 30-40 minutes or until golden brown.

Breakfast #23 (Continued)

BREAKFAST BAKE

Method

1. The night before, coat a loaf pan with vegetable spray.
2. Layer the pan with the bread, ham, peppers, onion, and cheese.
3. Mix egg, milk, and mustard. Pour over the layered ingredients.
4. Cover and refrigerate overnight. Next morning, place the pan in a cold oven and turn oven on to 350°.
5. Bake for 30-40 minutes or until brown and bubbly.

Dinner #23 (Continued)

HAWAIIAN KEBABS

Method

3. Remove chicken from marinade, reserving marinade. Alternate chicken, pineapple, green pepper, mushrooms, and tomatoes on eight skewers.
4. Grill over hot coals 20 minutes or until done, turning and basting frequently with marinade.

Dinner #24 (Continued)

CILANTRO SALSA

Yield: 4 servings/Serving size: 1/2 cup

Ingredients

2 tomatoes, diced
1 small cucumber, peeled and chopped
1 small red onion, diced
1/2 cup fresh cilantro leaves, chopped
Zest of 1 lime
1 small green pepper, diced
1-2 dashes hot sauce
Salt and pepper to taste

Method

1. Blend all ingredients to desired chunkiness and chill overnight.

Breakfast #25 (Continued)

CARROT-RAISIN MUFFIN

Method

1. Heat oven to 375°. Lightly grease muffin cups or use foil or paper baking cups.
2. Mix flours, baking powder, cinnamon, and salt in a large bowl.
3. Whisk eggs and sugar in another bowl. When smooth, whisk in buttermilk and oil.
4. Stir in carrots and raisins. Pour over flour mixture and fold in with a rubber spatula just until dry ingredients are moistened.
5. Scoop batter into muffin cups. Bake 20-25 minutes or until springy to the touch in the center. Turn out onto a rack.

Dinner #26 (Continued)

CHICKEN AND RICE BAKE

Method

1. Saute celery and onion in margarine.
2. Combine celery/onion mixture, parsley, rice, carrots, salt, and pepper.
3. Spoon mixture into 3-qt. shallow baking dish coated with vegetable spray.
4. Top with split chicken breasts.
5. Combine soup and milk. Pour over chicken. Bake 1 hour at 350° until chicken is tender.

Dinner #28 (Continued)

MUSHROOM SAUCE

Method

1. Melt butter. Add mushrooms. Saute until tender.
2. Add flour. Stir quickly, then add milk slowly. Cook over medium heat until thickened, stirring.

The snacks in this section are divided into three groups:

Each **60-calorie** snack equals	1 Fruit **OR** 1 Starch/Bread serving **OR** 2 Vegetable servings
Each **125-calorie** snack equals	1 Starch/Bread serving **AND** 1 Fat serving
Each **170-calorie** snack equals	1 Starch/Bread serving **AND** 1 Skim Milk **OR** 1 Meat serving

In some 170-calorie snacks, one Fruit serving has been used in place of either one of the Meat or one of the Starch/Bread servings.

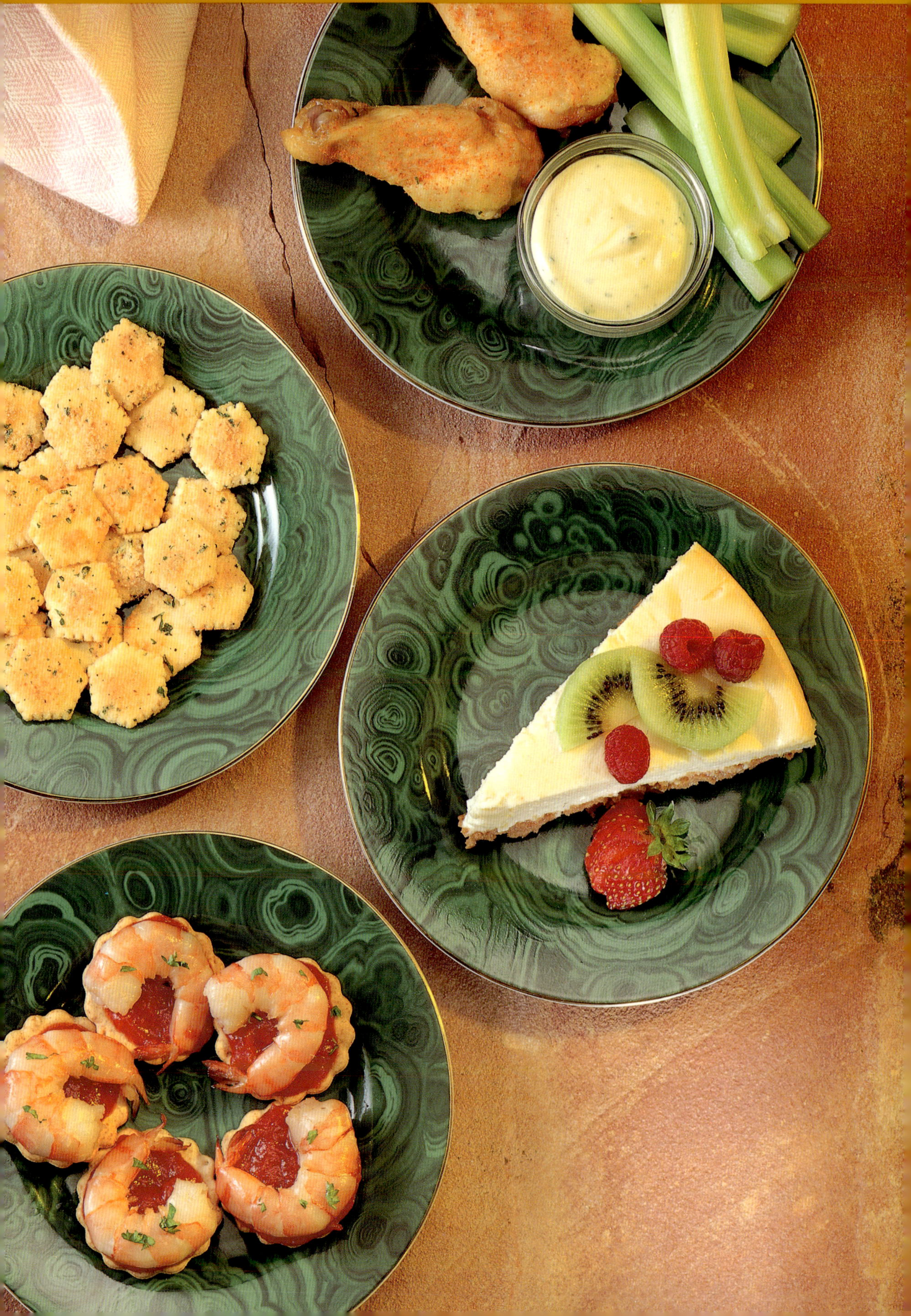

60 calories

1
1 English Pancake
(see Breakfast 17)

2
1 caramel popcorn cake

3
1 Apple Newton

4
1 cup carrot sticks with
1 Tbsp. Ranch dressing

5
1 cup puffed kashi

6
1/3 cup low-fat granola

7
3/4 cup donut seeds
(alias Cheerios)

8
1/2 cup STRAWBERRY WHIP

STRAWBERRY WHIP
Yield: 4 servings
Serving size: 3/4 cup

Ingredients
3-oz. box sugar-free gelatin
8 oz. nonfat plain yogurt
1 cup fresh strawberries

Method
1. Prepare gelatin according to instructions on package.
2. Beat hardened gelatin with rotary beater until frothy.
3. Add yogurt and beat gently until mixed.
4. Slice strawberries and stir into gelatin-yogurt mixture.
5. Freeze 10 minutes, then serve.

9
2 Cool 'n Creamy Orange Vanilla Crystal Light frozen dessert bars

10
7 dried apricot halves

11
4 Town House Whole Wheat Crackers

12
1 package (1/2 oz.) any flavor Skinny Munchies

13
1 package (0.66 oz.) any flavor Estee Snack Crisps

14
12 oz. any flavor Tropicana Twister Light

15
4 1/2 oz. any flavor DelMonte Fruit Naturals

16
2 Frookie ginger spice or mandarin orange chocolate chip cookies

17
2 Chico San rice cakes

18
1 Weight Watcher's chocolate fudge shake

19
Hot Mocha
(Mix 1 envelope hot cocoa mix with 1/4 tsp. instant regular or decaffeinated coffee and 1 Tbsp. evaporated skim milk powder.)

125 calories

1
No-Fat Steak Fries
(Slice a medium-large leftover baked potato with skin on into wedges and place on nonstick cookie sheet. Spray with butter-flavored nonstick vegetable cooking spray and broil until golden.)

2
1/3 cup low-fat cottage cheese
1/4 cup canned, drained pineapple chunks, packed in juice or water
1 Tbsp. raisins

3
Lite Sandwich
(Two slices of 50-calories-per-slice bread, 3/4 oz. low-fat cheese, tomato, and lettuce.)

4
Tortilla Chips
(Cut a 6-inch corn tortilla into triangles and broil until crisp. Top with 1/2 oz. grated mozzarella cheese.)

5
1 oz. dinner roll
3/4 oz. low-fat ham
1 tsp. reduced-calorie mayonnaise

6
Orange Cow
(Blend together 3/4 cup skim or 1% milk with 1/4-1/3 cup orange juice made from concentrate [not fresh] and drink immediately.)

7
1/2 cup any flavor Dreyers sugar-free low-fat dairy dessert

8
1 junior scoop in a cup of Baskin-Robbins sugar-free Low Lite & Luscious dairy dessert

9
1 nonalcoholic beer
1/2 oz. pretzels

10
1 slice low-fat lemon cheesecake **(see Lunch 13)**

11
1 Quaker Chewy granola bar

12
2 Fig Newtons

13
1 slice raisin toast
1/2 cup no-sugar-added apple juice

14
1/2 cup TUNISIAN EGGPLANT DIP on 6 crackers

TUNISIAN EGGPLANT DIP
Yield: 8 servings
Serving size: 1/2 cup

Ingredients

1 medium size onion, finely chopped
2-3 cloves of garlic, minced
2 Tbsp. olive oil
1/2 tsp. salt
1 large eggplant (peeled if desired), cut in 1-inch cubes
3 Tbsp. tomato paste
1/4 cup red wine vinegar
1 cup small green olives, pitted
1 6-oz. jar marinated artichoke hearts, drained and cut into 2-3 pieces each
Pinches of tarragon, basil, and oregano

Method

1. In large nonstick skillet, saute onion and garlic in oil with salt over medium heat until soft (5-8 minutes).
2. Add eggplant and cover. Cook 15-20 minutes until well done, stirring occasionally.
3. Stir in tomato paste and vinegar and heat to boiling.
4. Add olives and remove from heat.
5. Stir in artichokes and cool to room temperature.
6. Add herbs to taste.

15
16 Frookie Funky Monkies

16
12 Frookie Animal Crackers

17
7 1/2 oz. microwave Hormel Clam Chowder

18
1 oz. (about 14) FritoLay Sun Chips

19
1 sugar-free Eskimo Pie

170 calories

1
2 Tbsp. sunflower seeds
3 Tbsp. raisins

2
24 OYSTER HORS D'OEUVRES
(Mix 24 oyster crackers with 1 Tbsp. melted margarine. Sprinkle with a powdered low-calorie Ranch salad dressing. Broil until browned.)

3
1 hard boiled egg
2 slices "lite" wheat bread
1 tsp. reduced-calorie mayonnaise

4
1 cup Lentil Soup
(see Lunch 8)

5
1/2 bagel
1 Tbsp. peanut butter
1 tsp. artificially sweetened jelly

6
2 pear halves, canned in juice or water
1/3 cup cottage cheese
1 Tbsp. raisins

7
1/2 English muffin
1/4 cup egg substitute scrambled with
1 Tbsp. reduced-calorie margarine and
1 oz. low-fat ham chunks

8
3/4 cup PEACHY RICE PUDDING
(see Lunch 19)

9
1/4 Veggie Pizza
(see Lunch 15)

10
3/4 cup FRUIT CRISP
(see Dinner 13)

11
2 chicken wings
1 Tbsp. low-fat Ranch dressing dip
1 cup celery sticks

12
Milkshake
(Blend 1 cup skim or 1% milk with 1/2 cup sugar-free frozen yogurt.)

13
1 oz. carpaccio (raw salmon, available at a deli)
1/2 bagel

14
4 peanut butter/cheese crackers

15
1/2 Quesadilla **(see Lunch 1)**

16
4 cups popcorn lightly sprayed with nonstick vegetable cooking spray and sprinkled with
2 Tbsp. Parmesan cheese

17
1/2 cup BREAD PUDDING
(see Dinner 17)

18
5 medium shrimp
5 crackers
1 Tbsp. cocktail sauce

19
1 poached egg
1 slice whole-wheat toast

20
1 PEACHY WHOLE-GRAIN COOKIE
8 oz. skim or 1% milk

PEACHY WHOLE-GRAIN COOKIES

Yield: 30 cookies
Serving size: 1 cookie

Ingredients

- 1 egg white
- 1/2 tsp. almond extract
- 1/3 cup margarine
- 3/8 cup sugar
- 3/8 cup packed brown sugar
- 3/4 cup whole-wheat flour
- 1/2 tsp. salt
- 1 tsp. baking powder
- 1 1/4 cup quick or regular oatmeal
- 3/4 cup peaches, diced
- 1/4 cup dates, chopped

Method

1. Beat egg white with extract, margarine, and sugars in mixing bowl.
2. Combine flour, salt, and baking powder. Add to egg mixture and mix well with electric mixer.
3. Stir in oatmeal, peaches, and dates.
4. Drop by rounded (not heaping) tablespoons onto nonstick cookie sheet.
5. Bake at 350° for 15 minutes or until golden.

Photo at right:
Old-Fashioned Pot Roast and Gravy

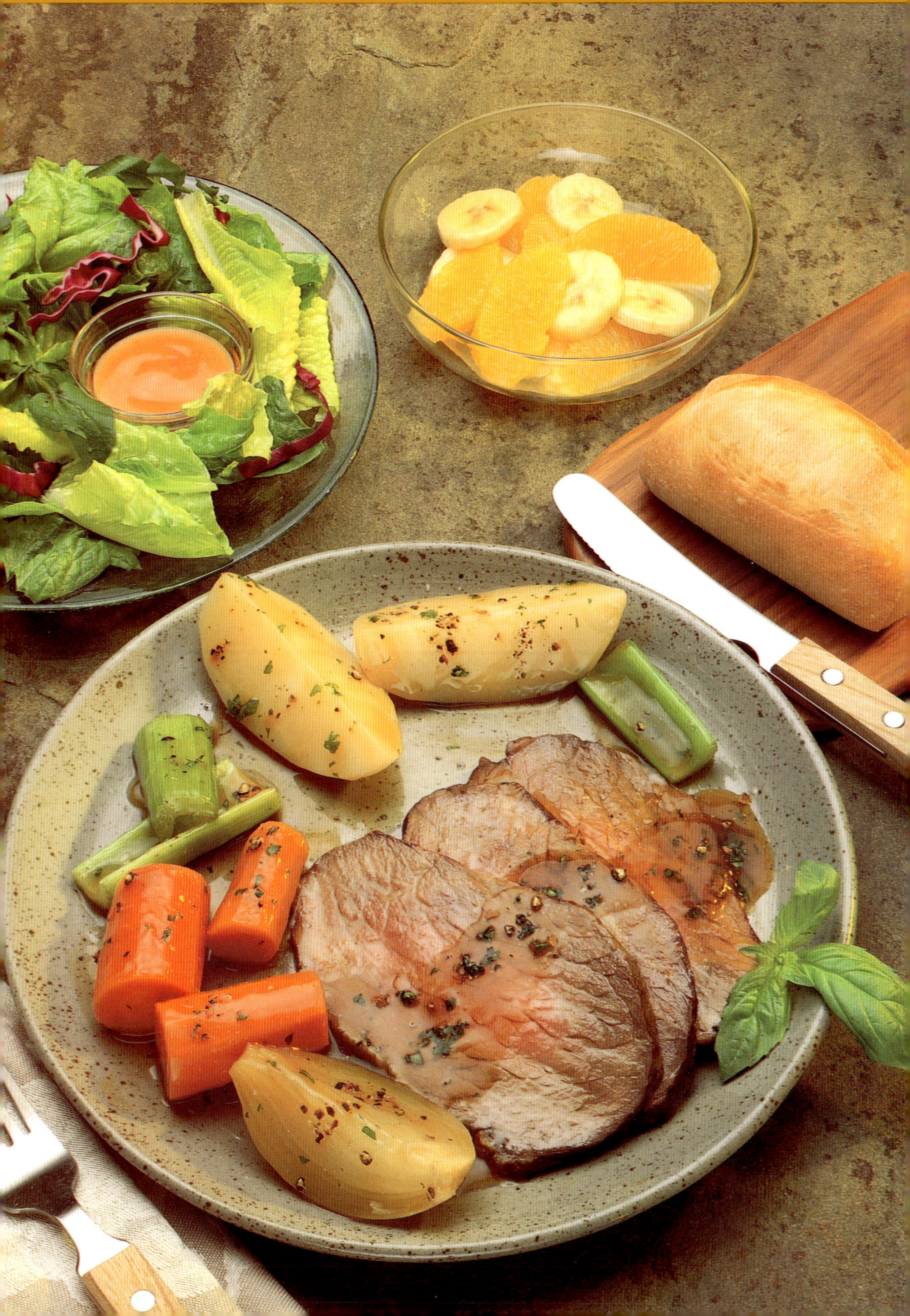

OLD-TIME FAMILY FAVORITES

Some dishes stand out among others. Their aromas and tastes bring back memories of good times with family and friends. Maybe it's your tradition to have pot roast on Sunday or a special meal unique to your cultural heritage when you gather together.

Many old-time family favorites tend to be higher in fat and calories than advised for healthy eating. Does this mean you have to give up the foods you love? No! You can still enjoy many, if not all, of your favorites. Some meals may be fine as they are, but adjusting the portion size you eat may be all that is needed. You can lower the fat in other dishes by using less fat in the preparation or by making a few easy substitutions. As you reduce the amount of fat, you automatically decrease the calories.

Take a good look at your favorite recipes, and try these tips to help lower fat and calories.

- Use 2 egg whites or 1/4 cup egg substitute to replace each whole egg in a recipe.
- Use skim or 1% milk in all recipes.
- Use part-skim cheeses to lower the fat and cholesterol content of your recipes. Part-skim cheeses should have 5 grams or less fat per ounce.
- Use lean meats that have 3 grams or less fat per ounce in your recipes; good choices are tenderloin, sirloin tip, and round steak.
- Remove chicken skin and trim excess fat from meats before using in a recipe.
- Use less margarine, butter, and oil when sauteing and panfrying. Use Teflon-coated skillets and nonstick vegetable cooking spray instead of adding oil.
- Skim fat from soups, stews, and broths by cooling them in the refrigerator, which hardens dissolved fats and causes them to rise to the surface.
- Adjust the serving size. Often the listed serving size is very large. A healthy portion contains 2 to 3 ounces of meat and 1/2 to 1 cup of starch.
- Top vegetable dishes with paprika, parsley, and other colorful seasonings rather than adding margarine, butter, or oil.
- Try using 1/4 the amount of margarine, butter, oil, mayonnaise, or shortening called for in baking.
- Use nonfat plain yogurt or fat-free sour cream instead of regular sour cream in recipes that are not heated.
- Stretch mayonnaise by mixing with skim milk or nonfat plain yogurt or try nonfat varieties of mayonnaise.
- Top casserole dishes with low-fat cracker crumbs instead of cheese, onion rings, bacon, potato chips, or croutons.
- Use less nuts and seeds in recipes. Six pecans have 150 calories!

For instance, do you love gravy? Your favorite recipe is probably too high in fat. But you can indulge in 2 oz. (4 Tbsp.) of the following gravy and consider it a free food:

HOMEMADE GRAVY

Yield: 8 servings/Serving size: 2 oz.

Ingredients

1 1/2 cups liquid (diluted fat-free juice from a roast or turkey; beef or chicken bouillon* granules or cubes; or combination)
1/2 cup water
3 Tbsp. cornstarch

Method

1. Dissolve cornstarch in water. Heat juice, then add cornstarch mixture.
2. Boil gently for 2 minutes, stirring constantly.

*Bouillon is high in sodium; use salt-free bouillon or soup base, or half regular and half salt-free.

We have prepared healthy versions of old-time family favorite dinners. We hope we have included your family's favorite meal.

• If the recipe makes too much for your family, consider halving the recipe (Cabbage Roll-Ups or Lamb Stew) or freezing extras as "planned-overs" (Meat Loaf or Pot Roast; see page 9).

• If you wish to eat extras as a lunch (menus are in dinner portions), omit 1 ounce of cooked meat (aim for 2 ounces total of cooked meat) and omit 1 fat serving, such as 1 teaspoon of margarine or 1 tablespoon of reduced-calorie dressing. For combination meals, such as Corned Beef Hash, about 3/4 cup makes a lunch portion.

2 1/2-inch slices of MEAT LOAF (2 x 4 inches)
1 cup boiled new potatoes
1 cup steamed zucchini
1 tsp. margarine
1 sliced tomato on bed of lettuce
1 Tbsp. Italian dressing

MEAT LOAF

Yield: 4 servings/Serving size: 2 1/2-inch slices

Ingredients

1/4 lb. ground pork
1 Tbsp. catsup
1 egg white
1/2 lb. extra lean ground beef
1/4 lb. ground veal
2 Tbsp. grated onion
2 Tbsp. skim milk
1/2 cup dried bread crumbs
Salt and pepper to taste

Method

1. Saute ground pork in a nonstick skillet, breaking it up until it is no longer pink.
2. Place pork in a colander and rinse with hot, then cold, water until it is cool.
3. Mix egg white and catsup, then add all ingredients and mix well.
4. Form into a loaf shape approximately 4 x 4 x 2 inches. Place on a rack in a Dutch oven and add 1/4 cup water.
5. Cover and bake at 350° for 40 minutes. Remove cover and baste with meat juices.
6. Increase oven heat to 400° and cook for 15 more minutes until slightly browned.

2

KIELBASA AND SAUERKRAUT
1 cup mashed potatoes
1 cup green beans
1/2 cup no-sugar-added applesauce

KIELBASA AND SAUERKRAUT

Yield: 1 serving

Ingredients

Nonstick vegetable cooking spray
3 oz. turkey kielbasa (about 4 inches long)
1 cup sauerkraut

Method

1. Heat a nonstick skillet coated with vegetable spray.
2. Cut kielbasa into 1- to 2-inch pieces and brown in the skillet.
3. In a colander, rinse sauerkraut in cold water; squeeze out excess water.
4. Add sauerkraut to browned kielbasa, adding additional water for juicy sauerkraut as desired.
5. Simmer covered until heated through.

3

2 RUSSIAN CABBAGE ROLL-UPS
3/4 cup no-sugar-added mandarin oranges, with
4 Tbsp. shredded coconut

RUSSIAN CABBAGE ROLL-UPS

Yield: 5 servings/Serving size: 2 roll-ups

Ingredients

1 lb. lean ground beef
1-2 minced onions
2 1/2 cups cooked rice
1/4 tsp. pepper
1 tsp. salt
Large head of green cabbage
10 3/4-oz. can tomato soup
6-oz. can tomato paste

Method

1. Mix together ground beef, onions, rice, and seasonings.
2. Remove any wilted leaves from cabbage head and scald entire head. As leaves begin to soften, remove them and place them hollow side up in a large pan.
3. When leaves are cool, fill with 1/4-1/2 cup of beef-rice mixture. Roll up cabbage leaves.
4. Mix together, tomato soup, tomato paste, and 2 cups water. Pour mixture over roll-ups. Cover pan and simmer on stove for 45 minutes.

4

1 serving
OLD-FASHIONED POT ROAST AND GRAVY with
1/2 cup potato
1 cup vegetables
Tossed salad
2 Tbsp. reduced-calorie dressing
1 dinner roll
1 tsp. margarine
1/4 banana and 1/2 orange, sliced

OLD-FASHIONED POT ROAST AND GRAVY

Yield: 8 servings/Serving size: 1/8 of recipe

Ingredients

3-lb. pot roast (rump, chuck, or shoulder cut)
1 tsp. Worcestershire sauce
1 tsp. instant beef bouillon granules
1/2 tsp. pepper
1/2 tsp. dried basil
4 medium potatoes, quartered
4 medium carrots, cut into chunks
2 medium onions, quartered
2 stalks celery, cut into chunks
3 Tbsp. cornstarch

Method

1. Trim excess fat from pot roast. Place meat in pressure cooker on rack. Add 1/2 cup water.
2. Bring to full pressure and cook 5 or 6 minutes. Reduce pressure by running cold water over cooker.
3. Remove meat to platter. Refrigerate. Pour liquid into a container and chill. When chilled, remove excess fat from meat and juice.
4. Return meat and juice to cooker and add vegetables and seasonings. Cook at full pressure for 10 minutes. Reduce pressure under cold running water.
5. Remove meat and vegetables to a platter and place in a warm (150°) oven.
6. Measure juice from cooker and add enough water to bring to 1 1/2 cups. Place juice in saucepan.
7. Blend cornstarch with 1/2 cup water until smooth. Add to saucepan. Boil gently about 2 minutes, stirring constantly, until gravy thickens.

5

1 serving SWISS STEAK
2/3 cup steamed white or brown rice
1/2 cup steamed crookneck squash
1/2 cup frozen yogurt

SWISS STEAK

Yield: 2 servings/Serving size: 1/2 recipe

Ingredients

8 oz. cube steak
1 Tbsp. flour
Salt and pepper to taste
Nonstick vegetable cooking spray
1/2 Tbsp. corn oil
8 oz. canned tomatoes
1/4 cup onions, chopped
1 celery stalk, chopped

Method

1. Cut steak into 2 equal portions. Combine flour, salt, and pepper and dredge steak in it.
2. Spray a medium skillet with vegetable spray. Heat oil in skillet and brown steak on both sides.
3. Add tomatoes, onions, and celery. Simmer over low heat about 30 minutes or until meat is tender.

6

1 serving LAMB STEW
2/3 cup cooked egg noodles
1/2 cup steamed asparagus
4 stewed prunes

LAMB STEW

Yield: 4 servings/Serving size: 1/4 recipe

Ingredients

14 oz. lean loin-cut lamb, cut into 1/2-inch cubes
2 Tbsp. flour
1 cup onion, chopped
1 clove garlic, crushed
Salt and pepper to taste
1 28-oz. can tomatoes
1 Tbsp. corn oil
1 bay leaf
1/2 cup beef broth

Method

1. Place cubed lamb in slow cooker. Add flour, salt, pepper, onions, and garlic. Mix thoroughly. Add remaining ingredients.
2. Cover and cook on low setting for 8-12 hours or on high setting for 3-4 hours. Season to taste.

7

1 serving CORNED BEEF HASH
1 slice toast with
1 tsp. reduced-calorie margarine
1/2 broiled tomato
1 cup mixed berries

CORNED BEEF HASH

Yield: 2 servings/Serving size: 1/2 recipe

Ingredients

4 oz. lean corned beef (from deli)
Nonstick vegetable cooking spray
2 tsp. margarine or butter
1/2 cup onion, chopped
1/2 medium bell pepper, chopped
1 cup potatoes, diced and cooked
2 medium eggs, poached
Paprika, salt, and pepper to taste

Method

1. Chop meat. Set aside.
2. Using a medium skillet that has been coated with vegetable spray, saute onions and pepper in margarine. Add potatoes and beef, and cook 8-10 minutes or until brown.
3. Divide hash into two portions. Nestle poached eggs in center of each portion. Sprinkle with paprika

8

1 serving YOGURT CHICKEN PAPRIKA
1/2 cup cooked egg noodles
1/2 cup steamed spinach
1 serving OLD-FASHIONED BANANA PUDDING

YOGURT CHICKEN PAPRIKA

Yield: 4 servings/Serving size: 1 breast half plus 1/4 cup sauce

Ingredients

1 1/2 cups onion, chopped
1 Tbsp. butter
1 Tbsp. paprika
4 chicken breast halves
1 cube chicken bouillon
1 Tbsp. cornstarch
1 cup (8 oz.) plain nonfat yogurt

Method

1. Saute onion in butter in large skillet. Blend in paprika. Add chicken and brown well.
2. Dissolve bouillon in 1 cup hot water and add to skillet. Cover and simmer 30-40 minutes until chicken is tender.
3. Dissolve cornstarch in 1 Tbsp. cold water. Blend into yogurt. Stir yogurt mixture into skillet and serve.

OLD-FASHIONED BANANA PUDDING

Yield: 6 servings/Serving size: 1/3 cup

Ingredients

1 oz. package sugar-free vanilla pudding
2 cups skim or 1% milk
12 vanilla wafers
2 large bananas, sliced

Method

1. Combine pudding mix and milk. Cook over medium heat, stirring frequently, until it boils, then remove from heat.
2. Place 2 cookies on bottom of each of six custard dishes. Alternate layers of bananas and pudding, starting and finishing with bananas.
3. Chill before serving.

9

1 serving APRICOT-GLAZED HAM
1/2 cup LIGHTLY SCALLOPED POTATOES
1/2 cup steamed green beans
1 slice "lite" wheat bread with
1 tsp. reduced-calorie margarine
1/2 cup sugar-free lemon gelatin with
1 Tbsp. whipped topping

APRICOT-GLAZED HAM

Yield: 4 servings/Serving size: 3 oz. ham and 1/4 cup glaze

Ingredients

1/2 cup orange juice
2 Tbsp. currants or raisins
1 cup juice-packed apricots, drained
1/4 tsp. ginger (optional)
12-oz. lean ham steak, fat trimmed

Method

1. Combine orange juice, currants or raisins, apricots, and ginger in a small saucepan. Cook over medium heat until thickened, about 8-10 minutes.
2. Place ham slice on baking pan. Pour sauce over ham and bake at 350° for about 20 minutes.

LIGHTLY SCALLOPED POTATOES

Yield: 8 servings/Serving size: 1/2 cup

Ingredients

1 clove garlic, diced
1/4 cup onion, diced
2 1/2 tsp. flour
6 oz. evaporated skim milk
3/4 cup skim milk
1/2 tsp. salt
1/4 tsp. red pepper
Nonstick vegetable cooking spray
4 1/2 cups (2 1/2 lb.) red potatoes, thinly sliced
1/2 cup reduced-fat cheddar or swiss cheese, shredded
1/3 cup Parmesan cheese

Method

1. In a nonstick saucepan, saute garlic and onion until tender. Add flour and mix well. Add evaporated milk, skim milk, salt, and pepper. Cook until slightly thickened, stirring constantly, about 2 minutes.
2. Alternate layers of potato, cheeses, and sauce in 2-qt. baking dish that has been coated with vegetable spray.
3. Bake at 350° for 45 minutes or until bubbly and golden brown. Let stand 20 minutes before serving.

INDEX TO RECIPES

This index lists items by the menu in which they appear. B = breakfast, L = lunch, and D = dinner. For example, the entry Bean Burrito, L14, indicates that the recipe is found in lunch 14.

Page numbers refer to the Snack or Old-Time Family Favorites sections of *Month of Meals 4*.

Now That We've Tickled Your Taste Buds, Dig Into Our Recipe-Packed Pantry of Cookbooks and Menu Planners

Month of Meals

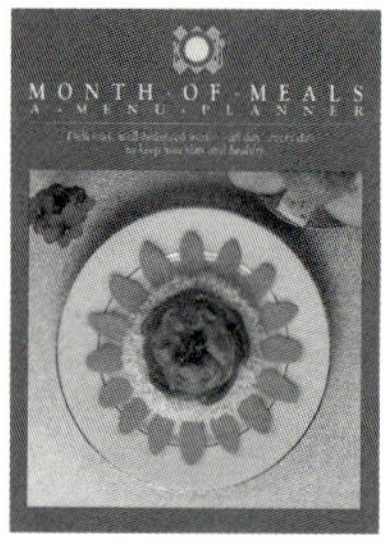

A "Special Occasion" section offers tips for brunches, holidays, parties, and restaurants to give you delicious dining options in most any setting. Oven Fried Fish, Sloppy Joes, Crab Cakes, many others. 57 pages. Spiral-bound. #CMPMOM
Member: $9.95
Nonmember: $12.50

Month of Meals 2

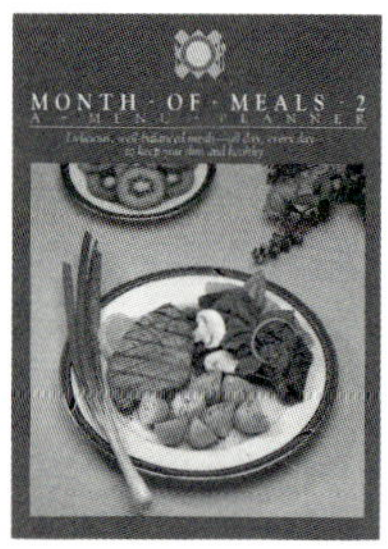

Tips and meal suggestions for Mexican, Italian, and Chinese restaurants are featured. Quick-to-fix and ethnic recipes are also included. Veal Piccata, Beef Burritos, Chop Suey, and more. 64 pages. Spiral-bound. #CMPMOM2
Member: $9.95
Nonmember: $12.50

Month of Meals 3

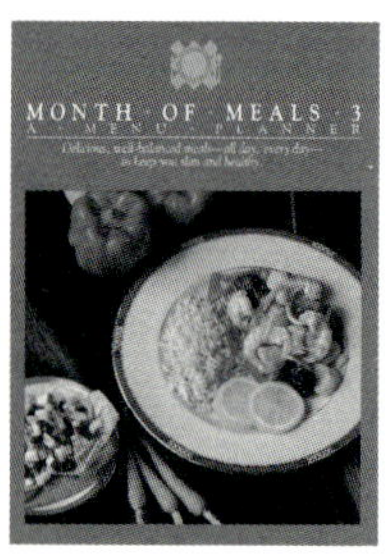

Special sections offer valuable tips: reading ingredient labels on packages; preparing meals for picnics and barbeques; planning meals when you're ill. Kentucky Fried Chicken, Stouffer's Macaroni and Cheese, many others. 72 pages. Spiral-bound. #CMPMOM3
Member: $9.95
Nonmember: $12.50

Month of Meals 4

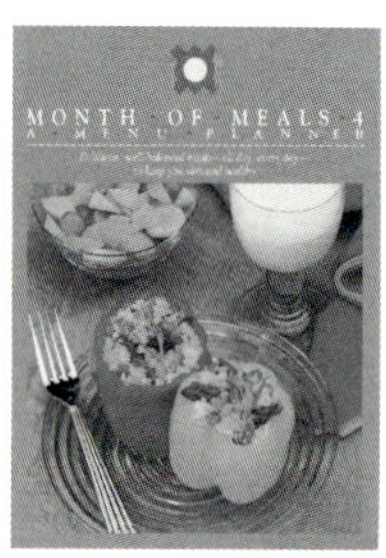

Hints for turning family-size meals into "planned overs" keep left-overs from going to waste. Meal plans for one or two people are featured. Oven Crispy Chicken, Beef Stroganoff, Meatloaf, Pot Roast, many others. 74 pages. Spiral-bound. #CMPMOM4
Member: $9.95
Nonmember: $12.50

NEW!
Coming in June, 1994
Month of Meals 5

A month's worth of fresh new meal plans with a special focus on vegetarian selections. #CMPMOM5
Member: $9.95 **Nonmember: $12.50**

SAVE 10%! Month of Meals Sets

Set of *Month of Meals* volumes 1-3. #CMPSET3
Member: $26.85
Nonmember: $33.75

Set of *Month of Meals* volumes 1-4. #CMPSET4
Member: $35.80
Nonmember: $45.00

Healthy HomeStyle Cookbook

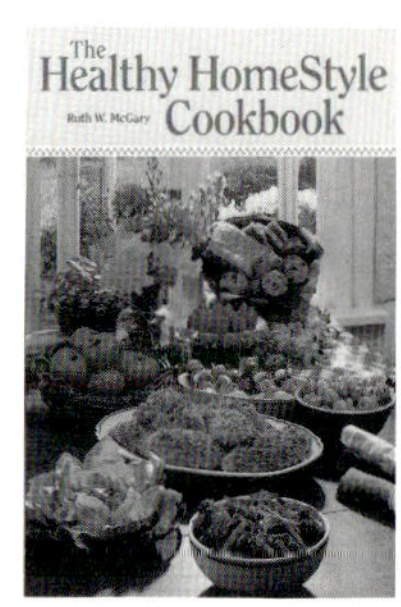

Come and get it! Here's home cooking at its best--and healthiest. More than 150 recipes low in fat, cholesterol, sugar, and calories. Try Dutch Apple Pancakes, Sweet and Sour Meatballs, Chicken Nuggets, many others. Includes energy- and time-saving tips for microwaving and freezing. "Lay-flat" binding allows hands-free reference to any recipe. 192 pages. Softcover. #CCBHHS
Member: $9.95 **Nonmember: $12.50**

Holiday Cookbook

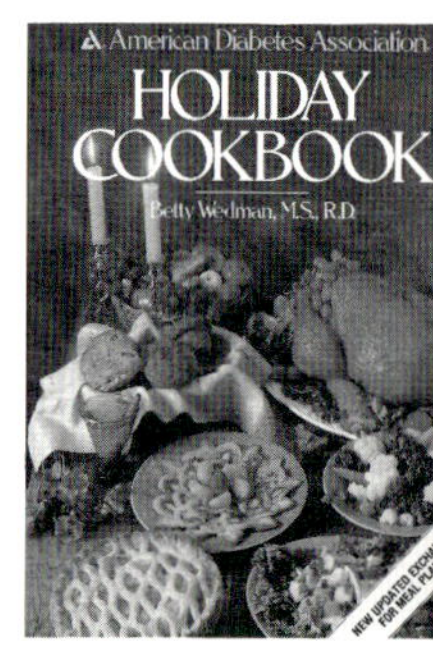

From Eggnog to Cranberry Rolls, our *Holiday Cookbook* will fill your table with tempting recipes from traditional Thanksgiving, Christmas, and Hannukah feasts to savory meal for any occasion. 219 pages. Hardcover. #CCBH
Member: $17.95
Nonmember: $19.95

Special Celebrations and Parties Cookbook

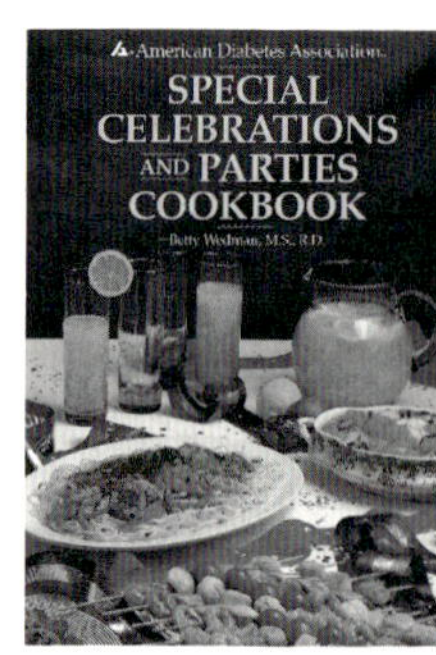

Cheesecake? Brownies? On MY diet? Yes! Whether it's a Fourth of July barbecue, Mother's Day brunch, or birthday bash, these recipes will tempt everyone's taste buds. 256 pages. Hardcover. #CCBSCP
Member: $17.95
Nomember: $19.95

SAVE 10%! Holiday Celebration Set

Includes *Holiday Cookbook* and *Special Celebrations & Parties Cookbook.* #CCBSET2
Member: $32.90 **Nonmember: $35.90**

Yes! Please send me the following:

____	copies of *Month of Meals*	$ ________
____	copies of *Month of Meals 2*	$ ________
____	copies of *Month of Meals 3*	$ ________
____	copies of *Month of Meals 4*	$ ________
____	copies of *Month of Meals 5*	$ ________
____	copies of *Month of Meals Set of 3*	$ ________
____	copies of *Month of Meals Set of 4*	$ ________
____	copies of *Healthy HomeStyle*	$ ________
____	copies of *Holiday Cookbook*	$ ________
____	copies of *Special Celebrations Cookbook*	$ ________
____	copies of *Holiday Celebrations Set*	$ ________
	Publications Subtotal................................	$ ________
	Virginia residents add 4.5% state sales tax.......	$ ________
	Add shipping & handling (see chart)..............	$ ________
	Add $15 for each international shipment..........	$ ________
	GRAND TOTAL.....................................	$ ________

Allow 2-3 weeks for shipment. There's an extra $3 charge for each additional shipping address. Prices are subject to change without notice.

Name ______________________________

Address ______________________________

City/State/Zip ______________________________

____ Payment enclosed (check or money order)

Charge my: ☐ MasterCard ☐ VISA ☐ Amex

Account Number ______________________________

Signature ____________________ Exp. Date ______

CH39401

Shipping & Handling Chart

Up to $30.00.......	add $3.00
$30.01-$50.00......	add $4.00
Above $50.00......	add 8%

Mail to:
American Diabetes Association
1970 Chain Bridge Road
McLean, VA 22109-0592

Yes! Please send me the following:

____	copies of *Month of Meals*	$ ________
____	copies of *Month of Meals 2*	$ ________
____	copies of *Month of Meals 3*	$ ________
____	copies of *Month of Meals 4*	$ ________
____	copies of *Month of Meals 5*	$ ________
____	copies of *Month of Meals Set of 3*	$ ________
____	copies of *Month of Meals Set of 4*	$ ________
____	copies of *Healthy HomeStyle*	$ ________
____	copies of *Holiday Cookbook*	$ ________
____	copies of *Special Celebrations Cookbook*	$ ________
____	copies of *Holiday Celebrations Set*	$ ________
	Publications Subtotal................................	$ ________
	Virginia residents add 4.5% state sales tax.......	$ ________
	Add shipping & handling (see chart)..............	$ ________
	Add $15 for each international shipment..........	$ ________
	GRAND TOTAL.....................................	$ ________

Allow 2-3 weeks for shipment. There's an extra $3 charge for each additional shipping address. Prices are subject to change without notice.

Name ______________________________

Address ______________________________

City/State/Zip ______________________________

____ Payment enclosed (check or money order)

Charge my: ☐ MasterCard ☐ VISA ☐ Amex

Account Number ______________________________

Signature ____________________ Exp. Date ______

CH39401

Shipping & Handling Chart

Up to $30.00.......	add $3.00
$30.01-$50.00......	add $4.00
Above $50.00......	add 8%

Mail to:
American Diabetes Association
1970 Chain Bridge Road
McLean, VA 22109-0592

Yes! Please send me the following:

____	copies of *Month of Meals*	$ ________
____	copies of *Month of Meals 2*	$ ________
____	copies of *Month of Meals 3*	$ ________
____	copies of *Month of Meals 4*	$ ________
____	copies of *Month of Meals 5*	$ ________
____	copies of *Month of Meals Set of 3*	$ ________
____	copies of *Month of Meals Set of 4*	$ ________
____	copies of *Healthy HomeStyle*	$ ________
____	copies of *Holiday Cookbook*	$ ________
____	copies of *Special Celebrations Cookbook*	$ ________
____	copies of *Holiday Celebrations Set*	$ ________
	Publications Subtotal................................	$ ________
	Virginia residents add 4.5% state sales tax.......	$ ________
	Add shipping & handling (see chart)..............	$ ________
	Add $15 for each international shipment..........	$ ________
	GRAND TOTAL.....................................	$ ________

Allow 2-3 weeks for shipment. There's an extra $3 charge for each additional shipping address. Prices are subject to change without notice.

Name ______________________________

Address ______________________________

City/State/Zip ______________________________

____ Payment enclosed (check or money order)

Charge my: ☐ MasterCard ☐ VISA ☐ Amex

Account Number ______________________________

Signature ____________________ Exp. Date ______

CH39401

Shipping & Handling Chart

Up to $30.00.......	add $3.00
$30.01-$50.00......	add $4.00
Above $50.00......	add 8%

Mail to:
American Diabetes Association
1970 Chain Bridge Road
McLean, VA 22109-0592

Order TOLL FREE!
1-800-232-3472
(Monday through Friday, 9:00 a.m. - 5 p.m. Eastern Time)
VISA, MasterCard, American Express accepted.

Our catalog is FREE. Just give us a call and we'll send you a copy.

Order TOLL FREE!
1-800-232-3472
(Monday through Friday, 9:00 a.m. - 5 p.m. Eastern Time)
VISA, MasterCard, American Express accepted.

Our catalog is FREE. Just give us a call and we'll send you a copy.

Order TOLL FREE!
1-800-232-3472
(Monday through Friday, 9:00 a.m. - 5 p.m. Eastern Time)
VISA, MasterCard, American Express accepted.

Our catalog is FREE. Just give us a call and we'll send you a copy.